f    Chinese    Medicine

Essentials of Chinese Medicine

# Materia Medica

**Dafang Zeng**

△△△ **Bridge** Publishing Group

## NOTICE

The contents of this publication are for educational purpose only. It is not intended to replace the diagnosis, treatments, prescriptions, and services of a trained practitioner or physician. The publisher and writers of this book have made every effort to confirm the accuracy of the information presented in accordance with current recommendations, regulations and standard practice at the time of publication. However, the authors, editors and publisher are not responsible for errors of omission or for any consequence from application of the information in this book and make no warranty, express or implied, with respect to the contents of the publication. Readers are advised to check the contents constantly for new and updated researches, clinical experiences, and government regulations might influence the practice of Chinese medicine and/or herbal therapy.

Printed in Hong Kong by Imago

**ISBN** 0-9728439-2-2 (Hardcover)

**Library of Congress Control Number**

2003100686

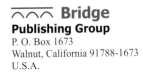

**Bridge
Publishing Group**
P. O. Box 1673
Walnut, California 91788-1673
U.S.A.

# Foreword

_Essentials of Chinese Medicine_ is a unified series consisting of multiple volumes. The first six volumes are <u>Fundamental Theories</u>, <u>Diagnosis</u>, <u>Materia Medica</u>, <u>Formulas</u>, <u>Acupuncture and Moxibustion,</u> and <u>Internal Medicine</u>. It is our intention to use concise, accurate and simple language to devote the essential knowledge of traditional Chinese medicine to our readers.

Consideration was taken into account to depict the characteristics of "essentials" when designing this series. "Essentials" signifies that each volume must clearly introduce to our readers the essence of the selected subject. In addition, the text is structured to be user-friendly for our readers to comprehend the contents. For that reason, this series was provided to the academy of Chinese medicine as a study tool for instructors and students.

This series is a collective achievement from a dedicated team of scholars. The principal author for each volume has extensive academic background and knowledge in the corresponding subject, and has been teaching in this field for decades. This qualification assures the scientific integrity and theoretical accuracy of the contents, as well as meets the practical needs of instructors and students from the oriental medical schools in the United States.

When organizing this series as a unity base on the systematic integrity of Chinese medical theories, we also emphasize the continuity among the subjects. We intend to minimize unnecessary repetitions or discontinuations in the contents among volumes. It is in our best interest to assure the consistency and accuracy in the interpretation and explanation of the Chinese medical terminology. We hope that _Essentials of Chinese Medicine_ will form the framework, and that by expanding and building upon it, a comprehensive set of textbooks on Chinese medicine will be completed.

As you read these books, we wish you find them helpful and stimulating.

**Bridge**
**Publishing Group**

# Preface

It has been more than twenty years since I began my teaching career after graduating from and working at the Beijing University of T.C.M. As an instructor, I often ask myself how I can help students comprehend Chinese medicine easily and clearly. During the last ten years teaching herbology in the United States, I further ask myself how to accurately explain the fundamental Chinese medical theories, the characteristics and properties of herbs. The primary purpose of writing this book is to accomplish these two missions.

There are 318 commonly used herbs in this book categorized into 19 chapters based on their therapeutic effects. The most common or the imperial herbs are presented in depth, each on a full page. Every herb is introduced by its unique characteristics and compared to its related herbs. Supplemental information is also provided in the comments section to clarify or to express some important concepts. Remarks and differentiations are provided at the end of each chapter.

Herbs are usually combined to bring out their therapeutic effects. It is from this perspective that this book was structured to incorporate all three major points (functions, indications and combinations) into one section. This structure can help students understand the application of herbs and be consistent in their learning process. Combining these points into one section is a unique feature of this book.

I have received great support from my family and my fellow colleagues. Without their dedication, this book will never be accomplished. I also want to thank the team at Bridge Publishing Group for their invaluable assistance. This book contains many accomplishments from authors and editors listed in the bibliography.

I am truly grateful to those who contribute to this book.

**Dafang Zeng**
Los Angeles
September 24, 2002

# Format Guide

## Zi Hua Di Ding .................... 1
*Herba Violae* ...................................... 2
*Bitter, acrid, cold; Heart, Liver* .................... 3

**[Characteristics]** With similar effects as Pu Gong Ying, Zi Hua Di Ding has a stronger effect in relieving toxicity. It is the primary herb for *Ding*.

**FUNCTIONS • INDICATIONS & MAJOR COMBINATIONS**

**Clear heat and relieve toxicity:** ............ 4
- *Ding*, erysipelas and any pattern of heat toxicity with sores and abscesses, such as breast abscess, etc. *+ Pu Gong Ying, Jin Yin Hua*  5

**[Dosage]** 10-30 g. Double the dose when using fresh form.

**[Comments]** *Ding*: Is a severe suppurative pathological condition that occurs on the surface of the body with acute and critical onset. Despite the insignificant swelling, it is deeply rooted into the body like a nail, known and pronounced as *Ding* in Chinese. Therefore, this pathological condition is named *Ding*.

**1. Pinyin Name:** According to the proper grammar of pinyin for the transliteration of the Chinese language, name of an herb should be in one word without a space between the syllables. For example, the correct pinyin for Zi Hua Di Ding should be Zihuadiding. However, to be consistent with the current practice of Chinese medicine in the United States, the former pinyin method of naming herbs is adopted in this book. In the future, the correct method of naming herbs will be standardized.

**2. Latin Pharmaceutical Name:** This book adopts the pharmaceutical names listed in Physicians' Desk Reference (PDR), 2000 edition, published by The People's Republic of China.

**3. Properties of herb and Channels entered.**

**4. Functions, Indications and Major Combinations:** This section lists the functions, indications and major combinations of individual herbs. The main signs and symptoms of pathological indications are described in the first few herbs of each chapter. This section lists the most common or classic combinations.

**5. Explanation of Chinese Pathological Terminology** (listed in *italics*)**:** For a full explanation, refer to the index to find the appropriate page, which also include the primary herb that treats each pathology.

# Table of Contents

# HERBS THAT
## Release the Exterior 1

Herbs in this category primarily dispel the exterior pathogenic factors and release the exterior conditions.

These herbs share some common characteristics such as acrid, dispersing and floating, and light in quality. They mainly enter the Lung channel to dispel the pathogenic factors from the superficial layers via sweating and are typically indicated for exterior patterns with aversion to cold, fever, headache, body ache, absence or presence of sweating, and floating pulse, etc. Some herbs from this category can also stop coughing and calm wheezing, promote urination and reduce edema, alleviate pain or vent rashes.

For exterior conditions of wind-cold or wind-heat, herbs that release the exterior are further subcategorized into acrid and warm herbs, acrid and cool herbs based on their unique properties and characteristics.

Acrid and dispersing herbs tend to injure the yin and exhaust the qi; therefore, excessive diaphoresis is not recommended. These herbs should be used with caution or are contraindicated in spontaneous sweating, night sweating, chronic sores and carbuncles, Painful Urinary Dysfunction or hemorrhaging. In addition, decoction over long periods of time may evaporate the volatile ingredients and can diminish their therapeutic effects.

# Ma Huang

*Ephedra* (handwritten)

*Herba Ephedrae*
*Acrid, slightly bitter, warm; Lung, Bladder*

**[Characteristics]** Characterized by its ability to disperse Lung qi, it opens the pores to induce sweating which releases the exterior. Therefore it is a powerful diaphoretic. Ma Huang disperses Lung qi to calm wheezing and coughing when the dispersion of Lung qi has been impaired. In addition, it also promotes urination.

### FUNCTIONS • INDICATIONS & MAJOR COMBINATIONS

**1. Induce sweating and release the exterior:**
- Exterior wind-cold excess with aversion to cold, no sweating, fever, headache, and tight floating pulse. *+ Gui Zhi*

**2. Disperse Lung qi and calm wheezing:**
- Coughing and wheezing due to impaired dispersion of Lung qi.
  - Wind-cold obstructing Lung qi. *+ Xing Ren, Gan Cao*
  - Cold fluids congested in the Lung. *+ Gan Jiang, Xi Xin*
  - Excess heat obstructed in the Lung. *+ Shi Gao, Xing Ren*

**3. Promote urination:**
- Edema on the upper body with exterior condition. *+ Bai Zhu*

**4. Wind-cold-damp Painful Obstruction and yin-type of gangrene.**

**[Dosage]** 1.5-10 g. Decoct first. Raw form is used for exterior conditions; honey-fried form is used for wheezing.

**[Precautions]** Contraindicated with spontaneous sweating due to exterior deficiency, night sweating due to yin deficiency, coughing and wheezing due to Kidney unable to grasp the qi. Use with caution in hypertension and arrhythmia.

**[Comments]** ❶ According to ancient saying, "Ma Huang is contraindicated in the presence of sweating". This restriction is meant for the formula, "Ma Huang Tang" only and not for the single herb, "Ma Huang". For example, the combination of Ma Huang with Shi Gao in "Ma Xing Shi Gan Tang" is used for excess heat obstructed in the Lung with profuse sweating. Ma Huang, in this combination, disperses Lung qi while Shi Gao clears heat as well as moderates the diaphoretic effect of Ma Huang. Consequently, heat will be cleared and sweating will be stopped.

❷ Ma Huang Gen, the root of Ma Huang, is categorized into herbs that stabilize and bind. For differentiation and application (p. 249).

❸ For coughing and wheezing, Ma Huang is commonly combined with Xing Ren for mutual assistance. For differentiation and application (p. 112).

# Gui Zhi

***Ramulus Cinnamomi*** Cinnamon (twigs)
***Acrid, sweet, warm; Heart, Lung, Bladder***

[Characteristics] Acrid to disperse, warm to unblock, it acts on both exterior and interior parts of the body. For exterior conditions, it works for exterior wind-cold excess or wind-cold deficiency. For interior conditions, its ability to warm and unblock yang qi can facilitate the flow of qi in the vessels, transform the qi, warm and unblock the channels.

**FUNCTIONS • INDICATIONS & MAJOR COMBINATIONS**

### 1. Induce sweating and release the exterior:
- Exterior wind-cold excess with aversion to cold, no sweating, fever, headache, tight and floating pulse. *+ Ma Huang*
- Exterior wind-cold deficiency with fever, aversion to wind, sweating, decelerating and floating pulse. *+ Bai Shao*

### 2. Warm and unblock the flow of yang qi:
- Wind-cold-damp Painful Obstruction. *+ Fu Zi*
- Dysfunction of the Bladder to transform qi with edema and dysuria. *+ Fu Ling, Bai Zhu*
- Chest Painful Obstruction. *+ Gua Lou, Xie Bai*
- Heart qi and blood deficiency with palpitation and intermittent knotted pulse. *+ Zhi Gan Cao*
- Dysmenorrhea and amenorrhea due to cold obstructing the blood vessels, and trauma induced pain. *+ Chuan Xiong, Dang Gui*

[Dosage] 3-10 g.

[Precautions] Contraindicated in yin deficiency with heat signs. Used with caution during pregnancy or excessive menstruation.

[Comments] ❶ Gui Zhi does not stop sweating when it is used alone. However, when combined with Bai Shao, a sour and astringent herb that can benefit the yin, they treat exterior wind-cold deficiency with sweating. This combination can harmonize nutritive and protective qi. When one disperses and the other contains, they expel the external pathogens and stop sweating.

❷ Gui Zhi is categorized into exterior releasing herbs for exterior wind-cold condition. Because of its ability to warm and unblock the flow of yang qi, its applications should not be limited to this category.

❸ Rou Gui, an herb that warms the interior, is also from the same plant, Cinnamon. For differentiation and application (p. 168).

**Acrid, Warm Herbs that Release the Exterior**

Chinese
Wild Ginger

# Xi Xin

*Herba Asari*

*Acrid, warm; Lung, Kidney*

**[Characteristics]** Releases the exterior and disperses cold. Characterized by its powerful acrid nature, it unblocks the nasal orifices and alleviates pain. It can also warm the interior and disperse internal cold, which is characterized by its ability to warm the Lung and transform cold congested fluids. It is therefore a primary herb to treat cold congested fluids hidden in the Lung.

| FUNCTIONS • INDICATIONS & MAJOR COMBINATIONS |
|---|
| **1. Release the exterior and disperse cold:** |
| • Exterior cold condition with headache and nasal congestion. *+ Fang Feng, Qiang Huo* |
| • Exterior cold condition and underlying yang deficiency manifesting with aversion to cold, fever and deep pulse. *+ Ma Huang, Fu Zi* |
| **2. Unblock the nasal orifices and alleviate pain:** |
| • *Bi Yuan* with nasal congestion, headache and runny nose. *+ Bo He, Xin Yi Hua* |
| • Wind-cold headache. *+ Chuan Xiong, Bai Zhi* |
| • Toothache due to blazing Stomach fire. *+ Shi Gao* |
| • Wind-cold Painful Obstruction. *+ Qiang Huo, Fang Feng* |
| **3. Warm the Lung and transform cold phlegm:** |
| • Cold congested fluids hidden in the Lung with wheezing and coughing up copious watery sputum. *+ Gan Jiang, Wu Wei Zi* |

**[Dosage]** 1-3 g. To open nasal orifices it is often powdered and inhaled directly into the nasal cavity. To stop pain it is powdered and applied externally.

**[Precautions]** Incompatible with Li Lu.

**[Comments] ❶** The ancient saying, "the dosage of Xi Xin does not exceed one Qian (approximately 3 g.)", stresses the importance of not exceeding the recommended dose of Xi Xin.

**❷** Xi Xin is categorized into herbs that warm the interior in traditional textbook. Such classification emphasizes its functions of entering the Kidney channel to warm the interior and disperse cold.

# Sheng Jiang   *Ginger*

*Rhizoma Zingiberis Recens*
*Acrid, warm; Lung, Spleen, Stomach*

**[Characteristics]** It has a mild effect to release the exterior and disperse cold; it is used for mild wind-cold or as an auxiliary herb in formulas. However, it is extremely effective in redirecting rebellious Stomach qi downward and is regarded as the imperial antiemetic to treat all patterns of vomiting.

| FUNCTIONS ● INDICATIONS & MAJOR COMBINATIONS |
|---|
| 1. **Release the exterior and disperse cold; often added as an auxiliary herb in formulas for exterior cold. Decoct this herb alone with black sugar for mild wind-cold conditions.**   *+ Da Zao* |
| 2. **Warm the middle burner and alleviate vomiting:**<br>• For vomiting due to various causes.<br>— Cold in the Stomach. *+ Ban Xia*<br>— Heat in the Stomach. *+ Huang Lian, Zhu Ru* |
| 3. **Warm the Lung and stop coughing:**<br>• Exterior wind-cold with coughing and copious sputum. *+ Chen Pi, Ban Xia* |
| 4. **Reduce toxicity of other herbs such as Ban Xia, Tian Nan Xing, Wu Tou, and also seafood.** |

**[Dosage]** 3-10 g. Slice and put into the decoction or grind to extract the juice.

**[Comments]** According to various processes, Sheng Jiang could be:

    **Sheng Jiang Zhi**, fresh ginger juice, is effective to stop vomiting, and can be used to process other herbs to increase their antiemetic effects, for example, Jiang Ban Xia and Jiang Zhu Ru.

    **Wei Jiang**, roasted fresh ginger, is effective in warming the middle burner, stopping nausea and diarrhea.

    **Gan Jiang**, dried ginger, is categorized into herbs that warm the interior. For differentiation and application (p. 169).

**[Addendum]**
## Sheng Jiang Pi
*Cortex Zingiberis Recens*
Acrid and cool, it specifically promotes urination and acts on the surface level; it is primarily used for *Pi Shui*. 3-10 g.

**Acrid, Warm Herbs that Release the Exterior**

*Perilla Leaf* # Zi Su Ye
*Folium Perillae*
*Acrid, warm; Lung, Spleen*

[Characteristics] Externally, it releases the exterior and disperses cold; internally, it promotes the movement of qi and expands the middle burner. It is frequently used for wind-cold conditions, especially when accompanied by cough or stifling sensation in the chest, fullness in the abdomen, and nausea or vomiting. It can also be used to treat Restless Fetus Syndromes.

| FUNCTIONS • INDICATIONS & MAJOR COMBINATIONS |
|---|
| **1. Release the exterior and disperse cold:** |
|   • Exterior wind-cold with cough. *+ Xing Ren, Qian Hu* |
|   • Exterior wind-cold with fullness in the abdomen and poor appetite. *+ Xiang Fu, Chen Pi* |
| **2. Promote the movement of qi and expand the middle burner:** |
|   • Spleen and Stomach qi stagnation with fullness in the abdomen, poor appetite, nausea and vomiting. *+ Ban Xia, Hou Po* |
|   • Morning sickness and restless fetus due to stagnant qi. *+ Sha Ren* |
| **3. Alleviate seafood poisoning.** |

[Dosage] 3-10 g. Should not be decocted for long periods of time.

[Comments] ❶ The alternative name is Su Ye.

❷ There are two more herbs from the same plant; Zi Su Geng is from the same category, and Su Zi is from another category of herbs that transform phlegm and stop coughing.

❸ Zi Su Ye releases the exterior and expands the middle; it is commonly combined with Huo Xiang. For differentiation and application (p. 83).

[Addendum]
## Zi Su Geng
### Caulis Perillae

It has the same properties as Zi Su Ye. With a stronger effect in promoting the movement of qi to harmonize the middle burner and calm the fetus, it is often used for stifling sensation and fullness in the chest and abdomen, and for Restless Fetus Syndromes. 6-10 g. Should not be decocted for long periods of time.

# Jing Jie  *Schizonepeta*

*Herba Schizonepetae*
*Acrid, slightly warm; Lung, Liver*

[Characteristics] Having the function of dispersing wind, it is useful for treating exterior wind-cold conditions. Since it is mild in temperature, it can also be used to treat exterior wind-heat. Charred form enters the blood level to stop bleeding.

| FUNCTIONS • INDICATIONS & MAJOR COMBINATIONS |
| --- |

### 1. Release the exterior and expel wind:
- Exterior wind-cold with aversion to cold, headache and body ache.
  *+ Fang Feng, Qiang Huo*
- Exterior wind-heat with fever, aversion to cold, headache and sore throat. *+ Lian Qiao, Bo He*
- Early stage of sores and ulcers accompanied by exterior conditions.
  — Wind-cold. *+ Qiang Huo, Chuan Xiong*
  — Wind-heat. *+ Jin Yin Hua, Lian Qiao*

### 2. Vent rashes and alleviate itching:
- The initial stage of measles with incomplete expression of the rash.
  *+ Bo He, Chan Tui*
- Wind rash or eczema with itching. *+ Chi Shao, Fang Feng*

### 3. To treat bleeding for blood in the stool, epistaxis, and other types of hemorrhaging, use the charred form.

[Dosage] 3-10 g. Not recommended to be cooked for long periods of time. The charred form stops bleeding.

[Comments] Usually, the entire herb is utilized; however, various forms are applicable according to the conditions and desired therapeutic effects:

**Jing Jie Sui**, the flower that has similar properties as Jing Jie, possesses a stronger diaphoretic effect compared to the entire herb.

**Jing Jie Tan**, the charred form that has lost the acrid and dispersing ability after being processed, exclusively astringes and stops bleeding.

**Acrid, Warm Herbs that Release the Exterior**

# Fang Feng

*Siler*

*Radix Saposhnikoviae*

*Acrid, sweet, slightly warm; Bladder, Liver, Spleen*

[Characteristics] Having the function of dispersing wind, it is useful for all wind conditions. Mild in temperature, it is used to treat patterns of wind-cold, wind-heat and wind-dampness. With its ability to extinguish wind and stop tremors, it can be used to treat tetanus.

| FUNCTIONS • INDICATIONS & MAJOR COMBINATIONS |
| --- |

### 1. Release the exterior and expel wind:
- Exterior wind-cold with headache, aversion to cold and body ache. *+ Jing Jie, Qian Hu*
- Exterior wind-heat with fever, aversion to cold, headache and sore throat. *+ Bo He, Jing Jie*
- Exterior wind-dampness with pain and heaviness of the head and body. *+ Qiang Huo*

### 2. Expel wind-dampness and alleviate pain:
- Wind-cold-damp Painful Obstruction with pain in the joints and cramps in the extremities. *+ Gui Zhi, Qiang Huo*

### 3. Extinguish wind and stop tremors:
- Tremors of the hands and feet or tetanus. *+ Tian Nan Xing, Tian Ma*

[Dosage] 3-10 g.         *Also stop diarrhea*

[Precautions] Contraindicated in blood deficiency with spasms, and yin deficiency with heat signs.

[Comments] ❶ Fang Feng enters the Spleen channel. It is noted for the function of "Reviving the Spleen". It can be used to raise Spleen yang and stop diarrhea (charred form), and is also useful in treating disharmony between the Liver and Spleen manifested in recurrent painful diarrhea.

❷ Herbs that dispel wind tend to be drying, yet Fang Feng is relatively moist and is known as "the moist herb in the wind-dispersing herb category". It expels external pathogens without harming the righteous qi.

# Xiang Ru  *Elsholtzia*

*Herba Moslae*
*Acrid, slightly warm; Lung, Stomach*

[Characteristics] Known as "Summer Ephadrae", its effects are similar to Ma Huang but milder. Exteriorly, it can induce sweating and release the exterior; interiorly, it can transform dampness and harmonize the middle burner. It is used for exterior conditions with summer-dampness.

| FUNCTIONS • INDICATIONS & MAJOR COMBINATIONS |
|---|
| **1. Induce sweating and release the exterior, transform dampness and harmonize the middle burner:**<br>• Wind-cold during the summer season with summer dampness, manifested as aversion to cold, fever, no sweating, abdominal pain, vomiting, diarrhea, thick and greasy tongue coating. *+ Bian Dou, Hou Po* |
| **2. Promote urination and reduce swelling for Spleen deficiency with edema.** w/ Bai Zhu |

[Dosage] 3-10 g.


# Qiang Huo  *Notopterygium*

*Rhizoma et Radix Notopterygii*
*Acrid, bitter, warm; Bladder, Kidney*

[Characteristics] Characterized by its ascending ability, it releases the exterior and expels wind-cold-damp to alleviate pain. Qiang Huo is generally used in Wind-cold-damp Painful Obstruction in the upper body. (Bi Syndrome)

| FUNCTIONS • INDICATIONS & MAJOR COMBINATIONS |
|---|
| **1. Release the exterior, disperse cold and alleviate pain:**<br>• Exterior wind-cold with aversion to cold, fever, headache and body ache. *+ Fang Feng, Bai Zhi* |
| **2. Expel wind-dampness, unblock painful obstruction and alleviate pain:**<br>• Wind-cold-damp Painful Obstruction, especially for the upper body.<br>*+ Fang Feng, Jiang Huang* |

[Dosage] 3-10 g.

[Comments] Qiang Huo and Du Huo have similar properties and effects; they are commonly combined together. For differentiation and application (p. 69).

*Ligusticum* **Gao Ben**

*Rhizoma Ligustici*
*Acrid, warm; Bladder*

[Characteristics] Expels wind and alleviates pain to <u>treat vertex headache</u>. It can also disperse wind-dampness and alleviate painful obstruction.

**FUNCTIONS • INDICATIONS & MAJOR COMBINATIONS**

**1. Release the exterior, disperse cold and alleviate pain:**
- Exterior wind-cold with headache, vertex headache or pain that radiates to the cheeks and teeth. *+ Chuan Xiong, Bai Zhi*

**2. Dispel wind-dampness and alleviate painful obstruction:**
- Wind-cold-damp Painful Obstruction. *+ Fang Feng, Qiang Huo*

[Dosage] 3-10 g.

[Precautions] Contraindicated in the cases of headache due to blood deficiency, and heat patterns.

*Angelica* **Bai Zhi**

*Radix Angelicae Dahuricae*
*Acrid, warm; Lung, Stomach*

[Characteristics] Characterized by dispersing wind-dampness and alleviating pain, it is <u>mainly used to treat Yang Brightness headache</u>, or frontal headache, and *Bi Yuan\** headache. It can also dry dampness, reduce swelling and expel pus.

**FUNCTIONS • INDICATIONS & MAJOR COMBINATIONS**

**1. Disperse cold and alleviate pain:**
- Exterior wind-cold with headache and nasal congestion.
  *+ Fang Feng, Qiang Huo*
- Yang Brightness headache located at the frontal and supraorbital areas. *+ Chuan Xiong, Fang Feng*
- *Bi Yuan* headache. *+ Cang Er Zi, Xin Yi Hua*

**2. Excessive vaginal discharge due to cold-dampness, sores and carbuncles.**

[Dosage] 3-10 g.

[Comments] *Bi Yuan\**: Manifested as nasal congestion with purulent nasal discharge and sinus related headache, resembles western concept of sinusitis. When this condition is unresolved and becomes chronic, hyponosmia could develop.

**Acrid, Warm Herbs that Release the Exterior**

# Cang Er Zi *Xanthium fruit*

*Fructus Xanthii*
*Acrid, bitter, warm, slightly toxic; Lung*

[Characteristics] Cang Er Zi is mainly used for *Bi Yuan* headache. It can also dispel wind-dampness and alleviate painful obstruction. It is slightly toxic.

| FUNCTIONS • INDICATIONS & MAJOR COMBINATIONS |
| --- |

**1. Unblock the nasal orifices:**
- *Bi Yuan* with headache, nasal congestion and nasal discharge. *+ Xin Yi Hua, Bai Zhi*

**2. Disperse wind-dampness and alleviate painful obstruction:**
- Wind-damp Painful Obstruction. *+ Wei Ling Xian, Rou Gui*

[Dosage] 3-10 g. Overdose may cause intoxication with nausea, vomiting, diarrhea, and/or abdominal pain.

[Comments] Cang Er Zi is categorized into herbs that dispel wind-dampness in some textbooks.


# Xin Yi Hua *Magnolia flower (bud)*

*Flos Magnoliae*
*Acrid, warm; Lung, Stomach*

[Characteristics] Dispels wind and unblocks the nasal orifices. It is the primary herb for treating *Bi Yuan*.

| FUNCTIONS • INDICATIONS & MAJOR COMBINATIONS |
| --- |

**Expel wind-cold and unblock the nasal orifices for *Bi Yuan* headache:**
- Cold type. *+ Xi Xin, Bai Zhi*
- Heat type. *+ Bo He, Huang Qin*

[Dosage] 3-10 g. Decoct the herb in gauze. This herb can be prepared as an ointment or aerosol for topical application or for nasal spray.

*M.nr* **Bo He**

*Herba Menthae*
*Acrid, cool; Lung, Liver*

**[Characteristics]** The light-weight, acrid and aromatic nature of Bo He helps it move and disperse the pathogenic factors. It mainly enters the Lung and Liver channels and it is also cool in nature. Exteriorly, it can disperse wind-heat from the Lung, clear the head and eyes, and vent rashes; interiorly, it can spread constrained Liver qi. Therefore it is commonly used for treating exterior wind-heat and Liver qi stagnation.

| FUNCTIONS • INDICATIONS & MAJOR COMBINATIONS |
|---|
| **1. Disperse wind-heat:** <br> • Exterior wind-heat condition and early stage of Warm-Febrile Disease with fever, slight aversion to cold and headache. *+ Jin Yin Hua, Lian Qiao* |
| **2. Clear the head and eyes, and benefit the throat:** <br> • Wind-heat with headache and red eyes. *+ Sang Ye, Ju Hua* <br> • Wind-heat with swollen sore throat. *+ Jie Geng, Sheng Gan Cao* |
| **3. Vent rashes:** <br> • The early stage of measles with incomplete expression of the rash or wind rash with itching. *+ Chan Tui, Niu Bang Zi* |
| **4. Spread constrained Liver qi:** <br> • Liver qi stagnation with hypochondriac distention and pain. *+ Bai Shao, Chai Hu* |

**[Dosage]** 3-10 g. Add to decoction towards the end. Use smaller dosage for treating Liver qi stagnation.

**[Comments]** The leaves of Bo He has a good diaphoretic effect to release the exterior, and the stem of Bo He is effective in spreading Liver qi.

# Sang Ye  *Mulberry leaf*

*Folium Mori*
*Bitter, sweet, cold; Lung, Liver*

[Characteristics] Light, ascending and floating in nature, it has a relatively mild effect in dispersing exterior wind-heat. With the primary action of clearing and draining heat from the Lung and Liver, this herb is commonly used for exterior wind-heat and Liver fire blazing up with red swollen painful eyes.

| FUNCTIONS • INDICATIONS & MAJOR COMBINATIONS |
| --- |
| **1. Disperse wind and clear heat:**<br>• Exterior wind-heat condition with fever, slight aversion to cold, sore throat and headache. *+ Ju Hua, Lian Qiao*<br>• Dry heat injuring the Lung with dry cough, scanty sputum, dry nose and throat. *+ Xing Ren, Bei Mu* |
| **2. Clear the Liver and brighten the eyes:**<br>• Liver fire blazing up with red swollen painful eyes. *+ Jue Ming Zi, Ju Hua*<br>• Liver yang rising with headache and dizziness. *+ Ju Hua, Gou Teng*<br>• Liver yin insufficiency with blurry vision. *+ Hei Zhi Ma* |
| **3. Cool the blood and stop bleeding for mild cases of hematemesis due to heat in the blood.** |

[Dosage] 3-10 g. Decoct and use as an external wash for eye problems.

[Comments] ❶ The alternative names are Dong Sang Ye and Shuang Sang Ye.

❷ In addition to Sang Ye, herbs related to the same plant are:

**Sang Zhi**, the newly grown twig of mulberry tree, is categorized into herbs that dispel wind-dampness.

**Sang Bai Pi**, the bark of mulberry root, is classified into herbs that transform phlegm and stop coughing.

**Sang Shen**, the mulberry, is categorized into herbs that tonify.

**Sang Ji Sheng**, the stem of an evergreen shrub that parasitizes on the mulberry tree, is categorized into herbs that dispel wind-dampness.

**Sang Piao Xiao**, the egg-case of mantis that is laid on the mulberry tree, is classified into herbs that stabalize and bind.

**Acrid, Cool Herbs that Release the Exterior**

_Chrysanthemum Flower_ **Ju Hua**

*Flos Chrysanthemi*
*Acrid, sweet, bitter, slightly cold; Liver, Lung*

[Characteristics] It has similar effects as Bo He and Sang Ye to disperse and clear wind-heat. Additionally, it nourishes the Liver and Kidney, as well as clears heat to relieve toxicity. This herb is commonly used for exterior wind-heat, Liver fire with red eyes, and heat toxicity with sores and abscesses.

**FUNCTIONS • INDICATIONS & MAJOR COMBINATIONS**

**1. Disperse wind and clear heat:**
- Exterior wind-heat condition with fever, slight aversion to cold and sore throat. *+ Sang Ye, Bo He*

**2. Clear the Liver and brighten the eyes:**
- Liver fire blazing up or wind-heat in the Liver channel with red swollen painful eyes. *+ Sang Ye, Xia Ku Cao*
- Liver and Kidney yin deficiency with blurry vision. *+ Gou Qi Zi, Di Huang*
- Liver yang rising with headache and dizziness. *+ Shi Jue Ming, Gou Teng*

[Dosage] 10-15 g.

[Comments] Two types of Ju Hua, grown from different geographic locations, are available for clinical applications:

      **Huang Ju Hua** (yellow), also recognized as Hang Ju Hua, is primarily used for dispersing wind and clearing heat.

      **Bai Ju Hua** (white), also known as Chu Ju Hua, mainly clears heat from the Liver and enhances visual acuity.

### [Addendum]
### Ye Ju Hua
*Flos Chrysanthemi Indici*
Bitter, acrid and slightly cold, it enters the Lung and Liver channels. Ye Ju Hua clears heat and relieves toxicity to mainly treat carbuncles, sores, swollen sore throat, and red swollen painful eyes. To treat sores, smash the fresh Ye Ju Hua; it can be used alone for topical application, or be decocted with Pu Gong Ying and Zi Hua Di Ding for oral administration. To treat red swollen painful eyes, it is often combined with Xia Ku Cao and Sang Ye. The decoction of Ye Ju Hua also can be used as an external wash for itchy skin. 10-20 g.

# Niu Bang Zi *burdock*

*Fructus Arctii*
*Acrid, bitter, cold; Lung, Stomach*

**[Characteristics]** When it vents and disperses, it also clears and drains. Disperses wind-heat as well as clears heat and relieves toxicity. This herb is often used in exterior wind-heat with cough and swollen sore throat.

**FUNCTIONS • INDICATIONS & MAJOR COMBINATIONS**

**1. Disperse wind-heat and benefit the throat:**
- Exterior wind-heat with cough, sputum that is difficult to expectorate, and swollen sore throat. *+ Bo He, Jie Geng*

**2. Clear heat, relieve toxicity and vent rashes:**
- The early stage of measles with incomplete expression of the rash or wind rash with itching. *+ Jin Yin Hua, Bo He*
- Heat toxicity with swollen sores and mumps. *+ Ban Lan Gen, Lian Qiao*

**[Dosage]** 3-10 g.

**[Precautions]** Contraindicated in diarrhea due to qi deficiency.

# Dan Dou Chi *Fermented Soy bean*

*Semen Sojae Preparatum*
*Acrid, sweet, slightly bitter, cold or warm; Lung, Stomach*

**[Characteristics]** Venting and dispersing exterior pathogenic factors for exterior conditions, it also disperses constrained heat in the chest and diaphragm.

**FUNCTIONS • INDICATIONS & MAJOR COMBINATIONS**

**1. Release the exterior and disperse pathogenic factors:**
- Exterior wind-cold. *+ Cong Bai*
- Exterior wind-heat. *+ Bo He*

**2. Clear heat and eliminate irritability:**
- Heat constrained in the chest and diaphragm with irritability, stifling sensation in the chest and insomnia. *+ Zhi Zi*

**[Dosage]** 10-15 g.

**[Comments]** Depending on which herb is used to process it, Dan Dou Chi could be cool or warm, and be used in either exterior cold or exterior heat condition.

*Cicada moulting* **Chan Tui**

*Periostracum Cicadae*
*Sweet, cold; Lung, Liver*

**[Characteristics]** This cold herb has the nature of lightness, ascending and floating. It is used for conditions of exterior wind-heat or Liver heat with exterior wind.

**FUNCTIONS • INDICATIONS & MAJOR COMBINATIONS**

**1. Disperse wind-heat:**
- Exterior wind-heat condition and early stage of Warm-Febrile Disease with fever, slight aversion to cold and headache. *+ Bo He, Lian Qiao*
- Lung heat with sore throat and hoarseness. *+ Jie Geng, Pang Da Hai*

**2. Vent rashes:**
- The early stage of measles with incomplete expression of the rash or wind rash with itching. *+ Ge Gen, Niu Bang Zi*

**3. Clear Liver heat and brighten the eyes:**
- Wind-heat attacking the Liver channel with blurry vision and red swollen painful teary eyes. *+ Ju Hua, Mu Zei*
- Childhood convulsion or night terrors, and tetanus.

**[Dosage]** 3-10 g.

**[Precautions]** Use with caution during pregnancy.

*Chaste tree fruit* **Man Jing Zi**

*Fructus Viticis*
*Acrid, bitter, cool; Bladder, Liver, Stomach*

**[Characteristics]** Dispersing wind-heat from the head and eyes, it is primarily used to treat headache and eye problems due to wind-heat.

**FUNCTIONS • INDICATIONS & MAJOR COMBINATIONS**

**1. Disperse wind-heat:**
- Exterior wind-heat with headache. *+ Fang Feng, Chuan Xiong*

**2. Clear the head and eyes:**
- Wind-heat disturbing upward with red swollen painful teary eyes. *+ Ju Hua, Chan Tui*

**3. Used for Wind-dampness Painful Obstruction.**

**[Dosage]** 6-15 g.

# Chai Hu Bupleurum

*Radix Bupleuri*
*Bitter, acrid, slightly cold; Liver, Gallbladder, Pericardium, Triple Burner*

**[Characteristics]** As an effective antipyretic, Chai Hu is the imperial herb for Lesser Yang Stage Disorder because of its ability to vent and disperse the pathogenic factors to treat alternating chills and fever. It is also the primary herb for constrained Liver disorder because of its ability to spread and soothe the constrained Liver qi. Moreover, it raises the yang to lift sunken qi.

| FUNCTIONS • INDICATIONS & MAJOR COMBINATIONS |
|---|
| **1. Vent the exterior to disperse heat:** |
| • Pathogenic factors trapped in lesser yang stage with alternating chills and fever, distention in the chest and hypochondriac regions, bitter taste in the mouth, dry throat, vertigo and irritability. *+ Huang Qin* |
| • Unresolved exterior pathogenic factors that are constrained internally and have transformed into heat with increasing fever and decreasing chills. *+ Ge Gen* |
| **2. Spread Liver qi and relieve the constraint:** |
| • Constrained Liver qi with distention and pain at the hypochondriac regions, irregular menstruation and dysmenorrhea. *+ Dang Gui, Bai Shao* |
| **3. Raise yang qi and lift sunken qi:** |
| • Deficient and prolapsed qi with weakness, shortness of breath, prolapse disorders, chronic diarrhea and chronic dysentery disorder. *+ Sheng Ma, Huang Qi* |

**[Dosage]** 3-10 g.

**[Precautions]** Contraindicated in yin deficiency with yang rising.

**[Comments]** ❶ Chai Hu is the imperial herb for Lesser Yang Stage Disorder when it is combined with Huang Qin. In this combination, Chai Hu vents the pathogenic factors in lesser yang stage, while Huang Qin clears heat in lesser yang stage. Together, one disperses and the other drains.

❷ Chai Hu is the primary herb for constrained Liver disorder and is commonly combined with Dang Gui and Bai Shao. In this combination, Chai Hu spreads Liver Qi, Dang Gui nourishes Liver blood, and Bai Shao preserves Liver yin. When Liver has sufficient yin and blood, Liver qi then flows smoothly.

❸ Injectable preparation of Chai Hu has a potent antipyretic effect for upper respiratory tract infections.

*Kuden* **Ge Gen**

*Radix Puerariae*
*Sweet, acrid, cool; Spleen, Stomach*

**[Characteristics]** Externally, it disperses the exterior pathogenic factors, suitable for exterior conditions with stiffness and tightness of the upper back and neck. Internally, it encourages the Stomach qi to generate the fluid and alleviate thirst. It also raises yang qi to vent rashes and to stop diarrhea.

| FUNCTIONS • INDICATIONS & MAJOR COMBINATIONS |
|---|
| **1. Disperse exterior pathogenic factors:**<br>• Exterior wind-cold with aversion to cold, fever, no sweat, stiffness and tightness of the upper back and neck. *+ Ma Huang, Gui Zhi*<br>• Unresolved exterior pathogenic factors that are constrained internally and have transformed into heat with increasing fever and decreasing chills. *+ Chai Hu, Huang Qin* |
| **2. Raise yang qi to vent rashes:**<br>• The early stage of measles with fever, aversion to cold, and incomplete expression of the rash. *+ Sheng Ma* |
| **3. Raise yang qi to stop diarrhea:**<br>• Damp-heat dysentery disorder or diarrhea. *+ Huang Qin, Huang Lian* |
| **4. Generate fluid to alleviate thirst:**<br>• Warm-Febrile Disease with irritability and thirst or Wasting and Thirsting Disorder. *+ Mai Men Dong, Tian Hua Fen* |

**[Dosage]** 10-20 g. Roasted form is for diarrhea.

**[Comments]** In modern application, the combination of Ge Gen and antihypertensive agents is used to treat hypertensive encephalopathy.

# Sheng Ma *Black Cohosh?*

*Rhizoma Cimicifugae*
*Acrid, sweet, slightly cold; Lung, Spleen, Stomach, Large Intestine*

**[Characteristics]** With relatively milder effect in dispersing and releasing the exterior, Sheng Ma is extremely effective in raising yang qi and lifting sunken qi; it primarily treats deficient and prolapsed qi. It also drains heat and relieves toxicity; it is used to treat patterns associated with heat toxicity.

| FUNCTIONS • INDICATIONS & MAJOR COMBINATIONS |
|---|
| **1. Release the exterior and disperse heat:** |
| • Exterior wind-heat with headache or the early stage of measles with incomplete expression of the rash. *+ Ge Gen* |
| • Measles with severe heat toxicity. *+ Zi Cao, Niu Bang Zi* |
| **2. Raise yang qi and lift sunken qi:** |
| • Deficient and prolapsed qi with weakness, shortness of breath, prolapsed disorders, chronic diarrhea and chronic dysentery disorder. *+ Chai Hu, Huang Qi* |
| • Qi deficiency unable to control the blood with Gushing and Leaking Syndromes. *+ Huang Qi, Dang Gui* |
| **3. Clear heat and relieve toxicity:** |
| • Yang brightness excess heat with headache, swollen and painful gum, sores in the mouth and tongue. *+ Huang Lian, Sheng Di Huang* |
| • Wind-heat ascending and attacking upward with swollen sore throat. *+ Jie Geng, Xuan Shen* |
| • Heat toxicity with sores and carbuncles. *+ Jin Yin Hua, Pu Gong Ying* |

**[Dosage]** 3-10 g. Honey-fried form raises the yang and lifts sunken qi.

**[Precautions]** Contraindicated in the conditions of excess above and deficiency below, and complete expression of measles.

**Acrid, Cool Herbs that Release the Exterior**

## [Remarks & Differentiations]

### Ma Huang — Gui Zhi

|   | Ma Huang | Gui Zhi |
|---|---|---|
| C | Induce sweating to release the exterior. Combined for mutual reinforcement for exterior wind-cold. | |
| D | • Powerful diaphoretic for exterior wind-cold excess only.<br>• Disperses Lung qi to calm wheezing for impaired function of Lung qi to disperse and descend.<br>• Disperses Lung qi to promote urination for edema. | • For both exterior wind-cold excess and deficiency.<br>• Warms and unblocks the flow of yang qi for cold obstruction in the meridians and blood vessels.<br>• Warms yang qi to promote urination for edema. |

### Ma Huang — Xi Xin

|   | Ma Huang | Xi Xin |
|---|---|---|
| C | Disperse exterior wind-cold. | |
| D | • Strongly disperses exterior cold and induces sweating.<br>• Disperses Lung qi to calm wheezing. | • Mildly disperses exterior cold and induces sweating. Also searches and dispels internal cold.<br>• Warms the Lung and transforms cold-phlegm to calm wheezing.<br>• Unblocks the nasal orifices, and alleviates pain. |

### Jing Jie — Fang Feng

|   | Jing Jie | Fang Feng |
|---|---|---|
| C | Acrid to disperse wind, mild in temperature. Treat both exterior wind-cold and exterior wind-heat. | |
| D | • Charred to stop bleeding. | • Expels dampness and alleviates pain.<br>• Extinguishes wind to stop tremors. |

## Bai Zhi — Qiang Huo — Gao Ben

| | Bai Zhi | Qiang Huo | Gao Ben |
|---|---|---|---|
| **C** | Disperse cold, release the exterior and alleviate pain. | | |
| **D** | • *Bi Yuan* or Yang Brightness headache where the pain is located at the frontal or supraorbital region. | • Pain at the upper half of the body. | • Vertex headache. |

## Bo He — Sang Ye — Ju Hua

| | Bo He | Sang Ye | Ju Hua |
|---|---|---|---|
| **C** | Entering the Lung channel to disperse exterior wind-heat. Entering the Liver channel to clear Liver heat and brighten the eyes. | | |
| **D** | • Strongly acrid to disperse. • Spreads the constrained Liver qi for Liver qi stagnation. | • Also bitter to drain heat. • For Liver fire blazing upward or Lung dryness with cough. | • Also sweet to nourish the Liver and Kidney. • For Liver and Kidney yin deficiency with blurry vision or Liver yang rising. |

## Chai Hu — Ge Gen — Sheng Ma

| | Chai Hu | Ge Gen | Sheng Ma |
|---|---|---|---|
| **C** | Disperse the exterior pathogenic factors for exterior wind-heat. Raise yang qi and lift the prolapse for deficient and sunken qi. | | |
| **D** | • Imperial herb for Lesser Yang Stage Disorder.<br><br>• Spreads Liver qi and relieves the constraint. | • Effectively treats exterior conditions with stiffness and tightness of the upper back and neck. • Generates fluid to alleviate thirst, and raises yang qi to stop diarrhea. | • Less potent in releasing the exterior, extremely effective in raising yang qi. • Clears heat and relieves toxicity. |

# HERBS THAT
## Clear Heat                                            2

They are cold in nature, and primarily clear and drain heat internally. Herbs from this category have three main objectives: clear heat and drain fire, cool the blood and relieve toxicity, and eliminate deficient heat. Most of these herbs are used for treating Warm-Febrile Disease in which the heat is lodged in the qi, nutritive or blood level. Toxic swellings, sores or carbuncles, and yin deficiency with heat are conditions that can also be treated with herbs that clear heat.

Based on their various natures and applications for different conditions, they are further divided into five subcategories: (1) herbs that clear heat and drain fire, (2) herbs that clear heat and cool the blood, (3) herbs that clear heat and dry dampness, (4) herbs that clear heat and relieve toxicity, and (5) herbs that eliminate deficient heat.

The middle burner is highly susceptible to the cold nature from the herbs in this chapter and can easily be injured; therefore, use with caution in patients with Spleen and Stomach deficient cold. If the condition is complicated with yin deficiency, it is recommended to add some yin tonics to the prescription. This is because cold and bitter herbs can dry out body fluid and can cause further injury to the yin. These herbs are also contraindicated for use in condition of true cold with false heat.

_Gypsum_ # Shi Gao

_Gypsum Fibrosum_
_Acrid, sweet, very cold; Lung, Stomach_

**[Characteristics]** Acrid, sweet, and extremely cold, it enters the Lung and Stomach channels. Extremely cold to drain fire and acrid to disperse, Shi Gao disperses heat from the layer in between the skin and muscles externally. Internally, it clears fire from the Lung and Stomach. It is the primary herb for excess heat in either qi level or yang brightness stage, Lung heat with wheezing and coughing, and Stomach excess fire. Calcined form (Duan Shi Gao) has an astringent effect to promote healing and generate tissue.

**FUNCTIONS • INDICATIONS & MAJOR COMBINATIONS**

**1. Clear heat and drain fire, eliminate irritability and alleviate thirst:**
- Excess heat in yang brightness stage or qi level with high fever, profuse sweating, intense thirst, big and flooding pulse. _+ Zhi Mu_
- Warm-Febrile Disease accompanied by excess heat toxicity with high fever, dark purpura and petechia. _+ Xi Jiao, Xuan Shen_
- Heat lodged in the Lung and impaired dispersion of Lung qi with high fever, wheezing, coughing, stifling sensation in the chest and nasal flaring. _+ Ma Huang, Xing Ren_
- Excess Stomach fire with headache, toothache and swollen painful gum. _+ Sheng Di Huang, Zhi Mu_

**2. Powdered form of Duan Shi Gao is used to treat eczema, burn lesions and non-healing sores.**

**[Dosage]** 15-60 g. Crush and decoct first. Raw form clears heat and drains fire. Calcined form is for topical application only.

**[Precautions]** Contraindicated in Spleen and Stomach deficient cold.

**[Comments]** Shi Gao is an extremely cold herb that clears heat. It is also a mineral substance that is heavy and descends downward, therefore the primary herb for clearing heat and draining fire. Moreover, with the acrid nature that disperses, when combined with Ma Huang, they treat heat attacking the Lung; Ma Huang disperses Lung qi and Shi Gao clears Lung heat. With the acrid nature that also moves, when combined with Xi Xin, another typical acrid herb, they treat constrained Stomach fire with toothache and swollen painful gum.

# Zhi Mu *Anemarrhena*

*Rhizoma Anemarrhenae*
*Bitter, sweet, cold; Lung, Stomach, Kidney*

[**Characteristics**] Bitter and cold to drain heat, sweet and moist to augment the yin; Zhi Mu acts on the upper to clear Lung heat, the middle to drain Stomach fire, and the lower to drain *Xiang Huo*.\* Moreover, it nourishes yin of the Lung, Stomach and Kidney. It can be used for heat patterns of excess or deficiency.

### FUNCTIONS • INDICATIONS & MAJOR COMBINATIONS

**1. Clear heat and drain fire:**
- Excess heat in yang brightness stage or qi level with high fever, profuse sweating, intense thirst, big and flooding pulse. *+ Shi Gao*
- Lung heat with cough and yellow sticky sputum or Lung dryness due to yin deficiency with dry cough and scanty sputum. *+ Bei Mu*

**2. Nourish the yin and moisten dryness:**
- Liver and Kidney yin deficiency with heat signs manifested as Steaming Bone Disorder and night sweating. *+ Huang Bai*
- Wasting and Thirsting Disorder due to yin deficiency. *+ Tian Hua Fen, Wu Wei Zi*

[**Dosage**] 6-12 g. Fry with salt water to enhance the effects of nourishing yin and directing deficient fire downward; raw form is used for other purposes.

[**Precautions**] Not recommended in Spleen deficiency with loose stool.

[**Comments**] ❶ Even though a bitter and cold herb, Zhi Mu is sweet and moist in nature. It simultaneously nourishes the yin and clears heat. Clinically, it is often combined with Huang Bai, another bitter and cold herb, to treat yin deficiency with heat signs. From this perspective, Zhi Mu is very distinct from other bitter and cold herbs.

❷ *Xiang Huo*\*: Historically, explanations of *Xiang Huo* are inconsistent. Generally, it is believed that *Xiang Huo* originates from the Gate of Vitality, and is stored in the Kidney, Liver, and Gallbladder, etc. In normal situation, it warms and nourishes the entire body, and promotes the functions of all organs. In the case of Liver and Kidney yin deficiency, the stored *Xiang Huo* fails to be contained, resulting in pathological manifestations of yin deficiency with excessive fire, such as five palms heat, tidal fever and night sweating, dizziness, vertigo and tinnitus, nocturnal emission and premature ejaculation. The therapeutic effect is to drain "*Xiang Huo*" or to put out the fire. "*Xiang Huo*" therefore refers to its pathological excessive fire due to yin deficiency.

**Herbs that Clear Heat and Drain Fire**

*Heat in all 3 jiao*
*↓ via urine*

*Gardenia Fruit* # Zhi Zi

*Fructus Gardeniae*
*Bitter, cold; Heart, Liver, Lung, Stomach, Triple Burner*

[Characteristics] Bitter and cold in nature, it descends downward. Zhi Zi clears heat from the Heart, Lung, Stomach, Liver and Triple Burner by promoting urination. It is especially effective in clearing heat and eliminating irritability; it also cools the blood and relieves toxicity. It is commonly used in the cases of Warm-Febrile Disease with irritability, Heat-type of Painful Urinary Dysfunction, jaundice, and hemorrhaging due to heat that causes the blood to move recklessly.

### FUNCTIONS • INDICATIONS & MAJOR COMBINATIONS

**1. Drain fire and eliminate irritability:**
- Heat constrained in the chest and diaphragm with irritability, stifling sensation in the chest and insomnia. *+ Dan Dou Chi*
- Excess heat and fire toxicity in the Triple Burner with high fever and irritability or sores, abscesses and carbuncles. *+ Huang Qin, Huang Lian*

**2. Clear heat and drain dampness:**
- Damp-heat jaundice. *+ Yin Chen Hao, Da Huang*
- Damp-heat-type of Painful Urinary Dysfunction. *+ Che Qian Zi*

**3. Cool the blood and relieve toxicity:**
- Heat causing the blood to move recklessly with hematemesis and hematuria. *+ Bai Mao Gen, Sheng Di Huang*
- Heat toxicity with either sores and carbuncles, or swollen throat and red eyes. *+ Lian Qiao, Pu Gong Ying*

[Dosage] 3-10 g. Raw form is used to clear heat and relieve toxicity; fried form is used to cool the blood and stop bleeding.

[Precautions] Contraindicated in the case of Spleen deficiency with loose stool.

[Comments] ❶ The alternative names are Shan Zhi and Shan Zhi Zi.

❷ For clinical application, usually, the entire fruit is used. However, three other forms are availabe according to various conditions:

**Zhi Zi Pi**, the peel of the fruit, acts on the surface and clears heat from the superficial layers.

**Zhi Zi Ren**, the seed, acts on the interior and clears internal heat.

**Zhi Zi Tan**, the charred form, also known as Jiao Shan Zhi, enters the blood level to stop bleeding.

# Lu Gen   *Reed Rhicome*

*Rhizoma Phragmitis*
*Sweet, cold; Lung, Stomach*

**[Characteristics]** Lu Gen clears Lung heat to expel phlegm and eliminate purulent discharge; it clears Stomach heat to generate the fluid and alleviate thirst, and to stop vomiting. It also promotes urination.

**FUNCTIONS • INDICATIONS & MAJOR COMBINATIONS**

**1. Clear heat and generate the fluid:**
- Heat patterns where heat injures the fluid with fever, irritability and thirst. *+ Mai Men Dong, Tian Hua Fen*
- Lung heat cough with thick yellow sputum. *+ Huang Qin, Jie Geng*
- Lung abscess. *+ Yi Yi Ren, Yu Xing Cao*

**2. Clear heat and stop vomiting:**
- Stomach heat with vomiting and hiccup. *+ Zhu Ru*

**3. Clear heat and promote urination to treat Painful Urinary Dysfunction.**

**[Dosage]** 15-30 g. Fresh form has stronger effects on clearing heat and generating the fluid, and should double the dose.


# Zhu Ye   *Bamboo leaf*

*Herba Lophatheri*
*Sweet, bland, cold; Heart, Lung, Stomach, Small Intestine*

**[Characteristics]** In addition to clearing heat from the Lung and Stomach, Zhu Ye also enters the Heart channel; it clears heat from the Heart and eliminates irritability. It provides an outlet for heat to be drained by way of urination.

**FUNCTIONS • INDICATIONS & MAJOR COMBINATIONS**

**1. Clear heat and eliminate irritability:**
- Heat patterns with irritability and thirst. *+ Lu Gen, Mai Men Dong*
- Heart fire blazing up with sores in the mouth and tongue. *+ Mu Tong*

**2. Clear heat and promote urination:**
- Heart fire shifted to the Small Intestine or Heat-type of Painful Urinary Dysfunction. *+ Che Qian Zi, Sheng Di Huang*

**[Dosage]** 6-15 g.

**Herbs that Clear Heat and Drain Fire**

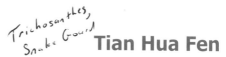

*Trichosanthes, Snake Gourd* **Tian Hua Fen**

*Radix Trichosanthis*
*Bitter, slightly sweet, cold; Lung, Stomach*

**[Characteristics]** Clears heat from the Lung and Stomach to nourish the yin and moisten dryness. Tian Hua Fen is suitable for fluid injury with irritability and thirst, and Lung dryness with dry cough. It also promotes purulent discharge.

**FUNCTIONS • INDICATIONS & MAJOR COMBINATIONS**

**1. Clear heat and generate the fluid:**
- Heat injuring the fluid with thirst. *+ Lu Gen, Mai Men Dong*
- Lung heat or Lung dryness with cough and viscous sputum or hemoptysis. *+ Bei Mu, Sang Bai Pi*

**2. Reduce swelling and promote purulent discharge:**
- Carbuncles, sores, ulcers and abscesses. *+ Jin Yin Hua, Bai Zhi*

**[Dosage]** 10-15 g.

**[Precautions]** Incompatible with Wu Tou. Contraindicated during pregnancy.

**[Comments]** ❶ The alternative name is Gua Lou Gen.

❷ Additionally, Gua Lou and Gua Lou Ren are also from the same plant. For differentiation and application (p. 108).


*Prunella flower* **Xia Ku Cao**

*Spica Prunellae*
*Bitter, acrid, cold; Liver, Gallbladder*

**[Characteristics]** Xia Ku Cao mainly enters the Liver channel. Characterized by its nature of bitter and cold, it clears and drains Liver fire; its acrid nature allows it to disperse and dissipate the nodules caused by constrained phlegm-fire.

**FUNCTIONS • INDICATIONS & MAJOR COMBINATIONS**

**1. Clear the Liver and drain fire:**
- Liver fire blazing up with headache, dizziness, red swollen and painful teary eyes. *+ Shi Jue Ming, Ju Hua*

**2. Clear heat and dissipate nodules:**
- Constrained phlegm-fire with goiter and scrofula. *+ Xuan Shen*

**[Dosage]** 10-15 g. Decoct or simmer to syrup-like consistency.

# Jue Ming Zi *Cassia Seed*

*Semen Cassiae*
*Sweet, bitter, slightly cold; Liver, Large Intestine*

[Characteristics] Sweet, bitter and slightly cold, it is also moist in nature. It enters the Liver channel to clear heat, drain fire, and brighten the eyes for eye problems due to wind-heat or Liver fire blazing up; it also enters the Large Intestine channel to moisten dryness, and unblock the obstruction of bowel movements.

| FUNCTIONS • INDICATIONS & MAJOR COMBINATIONS |
| --- |
| **1. Clear heat from the Liver and brighten the eyes:**<br>• Liver fire blazing up with red swollen painful eyes. *+ Xia Ku Cao, Zhi Zi*<br>• Wind-heat attacking upward with red and teary eyes. *+ Sang Ye, Ju Hua*<br>• Liver and Kidney yin deficiency with dull blurry vision. *+ Gou Qi Zi* |
| **2. Moisten the intestines and unblock the obstruction of bowel movements:**<br>• Intestinal dryness with constipation. Use alone in powdered form, or *+ Huo Ma Ren, Gua Lou Ren* |
| **3. Has the therapeutic effects to lower serum cholesterol for arteriosclerosis, and to reduce blood pressure for hypertension. Use prophylactically.** |

[Dosage] 10-15 g. Not recommended to decoct for long periods of time if this herb is used for constipation.

[Comments] ❶ The alternative name is Cao Jue Ming.

❷ Both Jue Ming Zi and Shi Jue Ming are important herbs for ophthalmological disorders. For differentiation and application (p. 187).

*Rhino horn* # Xi Jiao

*Cornu Rhinoceri*
*Bitter, salty, cold; Heart, Liver, Stomach*

[Characteristics] Salty and cold, Xi Jiao enters the blood level. It clears heat from the Heart, and relieves heat toxicity from the blood level. Xi Jiao is the primary herb in the cases of heat lodged in the nutritive and blood level of Warm-Febrile Disease. It is used for high fever, loss of consciousness, convulsions and epilepsy, and bleeding due to heat causing the blood to move recklessly.

**FUNCTIONS • INDICATIONS & MAJOR COMBINATIONS**

**1. Clear heat from the Heart, relieve toxicity, and arrest convulsions:**
- Heat lodged in the nutritive and blood level of Warm-Febrile Disease with fever worse at night, irritability and restlessness, loss of consciousness and delirium. *+ Huang Lian, Xuan Shen*
- Warm-Febrile Disease with high fever, irritability, convulsions and epilepsy. *+ Ling Yang Jiao*
- Warm-Febrile Disease accompanied by excess heat toxicity with high fever, dark purpura and petechia. *+ Shi Gao, Xuan Shen*

**2. Cool the blood and stop bleeding:**
- Heat causing the blood to move recklessly with hematemesis, subcutaneous and mucosa hemorrhage. *+ Sheng Di Huang, Chi Shao*

[Dosage] 1.5-6 g. File to powder and take with warm water or decoction; or grind to juice; or add to pill.

[Precautions] Antagonized with Chuan Wu and Cao Wu. Xi Jiao should be used with caution during pregnancy.

[Comments] Xi Jiao is commonly used for Warm-Febrile Disease with high fever and loss of consciousness; for extreme heat generating internal wind, it is often combined with Ling Yang Jiao. For differentiation and application (p. 191).

[Addendum]
**Shui Niu Jiao** *Water Buffalo horn*
*Cornu Bubali*
Salty and cold, it clears heat, cools the blood, and relieves toxicity. It is used for high fever, loss of consciousness, heat patterns with purpura and petechia, and extreme heat with hemorrhages. It has similar effects as Xi Jiao; currently, it is frequently used in place of Xi Jiao. Because of its milder effect, a larger dose is recommended. 15-30 g. Same preparations as Xi Jiao.

# Sheng Di Huang *Rehmannia*

*Radix Rehmanniae*
*Sweet, bitter, cold; Heart, Liver, Kidney*

[Characteristics] It is the primary herb for clearing heat and cooling the blood. Furthermore, sweet, cold, moist and juicy consistency, it nourishes the yin and generates the fluid. It is a common herb for excess heat in the blood level, yin deficiency with heat, and yin deficiency patterns of any yin or yang organ.

| FUNCTIONS • INDICATIONS & MAJOR COMBINATIONS |
| --- |
| **1. Clear heat and cool the blood:**<br>• Heat lodged in the nutritive and blood level of Warm-Febrile Disease with fever worse at night, irritability and restlessness, loss of consciousness and delirium. *+ Xi Jiao, Xuan Shen*<br>• Heat causing the blood to move recklessly with hematemesis, subcutaneous and mucosa hemorrhage. *+ Xi Jiao, Chi Shao* |
| **2. Nourish the yin and generate the fluid:**<br>• Patterns of heat with yin injury.<br>— Stomach yin insufficiency. *+ Mai Men Dong, Yu Zhu*<br>— Wasting and Thirsting Disorder. *+ Ge Gen, Tian Hua Fen*<br>— Intestinal dryness with constipation. *+ Mai Men Dong, Xuan Shen* |

[Dosage] 10-30 g. Double the dose when using fresh form.

[Precautions] Not recommended in the case of Spleen deficiency and excessive dampness with loose stool.

[Comments] ❶ The alternative name is Gan Di Huang.

❷ Fresh form is Xian Di Huang; honey-fried form is Shu Di Huang. For differentiation and application (p. 217).

❸ Sheng Di Huang is classified into the category of clearing heat and cooling the blood. However, recognizing its sweet and cold nature, moist and juicy consistency, one should realize that it can nourish the yin and generate the fluid. Therefore, for all patterns of yin deficiency, Sheng Di Huang is commonly combined with herbs that nourish the yin. Its application goes beyond its classification.

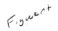
*Figwort*

# Xuan Shen

*Radix Scrophulariae*
*Salty, sweet, bitter, cold; Lung, Stomach, Kidney*

[Characteristics] Having similar effects as Sheng Di Huang, Xuan Shen can clear heat, cool the blood, nourish the yin and drain fire; moreover, as being salty and cold in nature, it has the effects to soften hardness, relieve toxicity and dissipate nodules. It is commonly used in the cases of heat lodged in the nutritive and blood level of Warm-Febrile Disease, yin deficiency with heat, scrofula and sores due to heat toxicity.

**FUNCTIONS • INDICATIONS & MAJOR COMBINATIONS**

### 1. Clear heat and generate the fluid:
- Heat lodged in the nutritive and blood level of Warm-Febrile Disease with fever worse at night, irritability and restlessness, loss of consciousness and delirium. *+ Xi Jiao, Sheng Di Huang*
- Excess heat toxicity with high fever, dark-red purpura and petechia. *+ Xi Jiao, Shi Gao*

### 2. Relieve toxicity and dissipate nodules:
- Exterior wind-heat with swollen sore throat. *+ Jie Geng, Lian Qiao*
- Fire toxicity with sores, carbuncles, ulcers and swelling. *+ Jin Yin Hua, Lian Qiao*
- Phlegm-fire with scrofula, goiter and other nodules on the neck. *+ Mu Li, Bei Mu*
- Sloughing gangrene. *+ Jin Yin Hua, Dang Gui*

[Dosage] 10-15 g.

[Precautions] Incompatible with Li Lu. Not recommended in Spleen deficiency with loose stool.

# Mu Dan Pi    Moutan

*Cortex Moutan*
*Bitter, acrid, slightly cold; Heart, Liver, Kidney*

[Characteristics] Mainly enters the Heart and Liver, or blood level. Mu Dan Pi clears heat, cools the blood, as well as invigorates the blood and dispels blood stasis. It is recognized by the characteristics of "cooling blood without leaving stasis, invigorating blood without disturbing the blood"; therefore, it is used for heat in the blood level or blood stasis due to heat consuming fluid in the blood.

## FUNCTIONS • INDICATIONS & MAJOR COMBINATIONS

### 1. Clear heat and cool the blood:
- Heat lodged in the blood level of Warm-Febrile Disease with dark purpura and petechia or heat causing the blood to move recklessly with hemorrhages. *+ Xi Jiao, Chi Shao*
- Late stage of Warm-Febrile Disease, heat lingering in the yin level with fever at night that recedes in the morning and absence of sweating as fever reduces. *+ Qing Hao, Bie Jia*

### 2. Invigorate the blood and dispel stasis:
- Blood stasis with dysmenorrhea and amenorrhea. *+ Tao Ren, Gui Zhi*
- Traumatic injuries with blood stasis and pain. *+ Ru Xiang, Mo Yao*

### 3. Cool the blood and reduce abscess:
- Toxic swelling, carbuncles and sores.
  — Dermal abscesses and sores. *+ Jin Yin Hua, Lian Qiao*
  — Intestinal abscess. *+ Da Huang, Tao Ren*

[Dosage] 6-10 g.

[Precautions] Not recommended in blood deficiency with cold, excessive menstruation and pregnancy.

*lithospermum*

# Zi Cao

*Radix Arnebiae seu Lithospermi*
*Sweet, cold; Heart, Liver*

[Characteristics] It cools the blood, invigorates the blood, as well as relieves toxicity and vents rashes.

**FUNCTIONS • INDICATIONS & MAJOR COMBINATIONS**

### 1. Cool the blood, invigorate the blood, and vent rashes:
- Warm-Febrile Disease with dark-red purpura and petechia, and measles with either incomplete expression of the rashes or dark-red rashes. *+ Chan Tui, Chi Shao*
- For preventing infection or to ease the symptoms of measles. *+ Sheng Gan Cao, Lu Dou*

### 2. Relieve fire toxicity for sores, abscesses, carbuncles, ulcers and toxic swelling or burn lesions. Use ointment for topical application.

[Dosage] 3-10 g.

[Precautions] Contraindicated in Spleen deficiency with loose stool.

# Huang Qin *Scutellaria*

*Radix Scutellariae*
*Bitter, cold; Lung, Stomach, Gallbladder, Large Intestine*

[Characteristics] Primarily clears heat and dries dampness. Huang Qin is especially effective in clearing heat from the Lung and upper burner; it also can stop bleeding and calm the fetus. It is mainly used for Lung heat cough, constrained heat in the upper burner, damp-heat diarrhea and dysentery, and Restless Fetus Syndromes.

| FUNCTIONS • INDICATIONS & MAJOR COMBINATIONS |
|---|

**1. Clear heat and dry dampness:**
- Damp-warm Febrile Disease with stifling sensation in the chest and yellow greasy tongue coating. *+ Hua Shi, Bai Dou Kou*
- Damp-heat jaundice. *+ Zhi Zi, Yin Chen Hao*
- Stomach and Large Intestine damp-heat causing diarrhea or dysentery disorder. *+ Huang Lian, Mu Xiang*
- Lower burner damp-heat with Urinary Painful Dysfunction. *+ Sheng Di Huang, Mu Tong*

**2. Clear heat, drain fire, and relieve toxicity:**
- Pathogenic factors trapped in the lesser yang stage with alternating chills and fever. *+ Chai Hu*
- Lung heat with cough and yellow sticky sputum. *+ Sang Bai Pi*
- Excess heat and fire toxicity in the Triple Burner with high fever and irritability or sores and abscesses, etc. *+ Huang Lian, Zhi Zi*

**3. Clear heat and stop bleeding:** *Huang Qin Tan*
- Heat causing the blood to move recklessly with hematemesis, hemoptysis, blood in the stool, subcutaneous and mucosa hemorrhage. *+ Sheng Di Huang, Bai Mao Gen*

**4. Clear heat and calm the fetus:**
- Restless Fetus Syndromes due to warm womb. *+ Bai Zu, Dang Gui*

[Dosage] 3-10 g. Raw to clear heat; fried to calm the fetus; charred to stop bleeding; fry with wine to clear heat from the upper burner.

[Precautions] Contraindicated in Spleen and Stomach deficient cold.

[Comments] Huang Qin primarily clears heat from the Lung and upper burner. Nevertheless, as indicated above, it is used to clear heat from any organ with appropriate combinations. Huang Qin is evidently an herb that clears heat with broad spectrum applications.

*Coptis* # Huang Lian

*Rhizoma Coptidis*
*Bitter, cold; Heart, Liver, Stomach, Large Intestine*

[Characteristics] Extremely bitter, cold, and drying in nature, it is especially effective in clearing Heart heat, draining Stomach fire and clearing damp-heat from the Stomach and intestines. Huang Lian is the primary herb for conditions of damp-heat, constrained fire, and heat toxicity. It is primarily used to treat Heart fire excess, Stomach fire excess, heat toxicity with sores and abscesses, damp-heat diarrhea and dysentery.

### FUNCTIONS • INDICATIONS & MAJOR COMBINATIONS

**1. Clear heat and dry dampness:**
- Stomach and Large Intestine damp-heat causing diarrhea or dysentery disorder. *+ Huang Qin, Mu Xiang*

**2. Drain fire and relieve toxicity:**
- Heat lodged in the nutritive and blood level of Warm-Febrile Disease with fever worse at night, irritability and restlessness, loss of consciousness and delirium. *+ Xi Jiao, Sheng Di Huang*
- Heart fire with irritability, insomnia, sores of the mouth and tongue. *+ Zhu Sha, Sheng Di Huang*
- Lack of communication between the Heart and Kidney with irritability and insomnia. *+ E Jiao*
- Stomach fire with bitter taste in the mouth, bad breath, vomiting and toothache. *+ Shi Gao, Zhu Ru*
- Excess heat and fire toxicity in the Triple Burner with high fever and irritability or sores and abscesses, etc. *+ Huang Qin, Zhi Zi*

**3. Clear and drain Liver fire to treat Liver fire invading the Stomach with vomiting, acid regurgitation and bitter taste in the mouth. Commonly** *+ Wu Zhu Yu*

[Dosage] 3-10 g. Fry with ginger juice to stop vomiting; fry with wine to relieve heat toxicity from the upper burner.

[Precautions] With its extremely bitter and cold nature, Huang Lian could injure the Spleen and Stomach with overdose or with long-term use. Contraindicated in the cases of Stomach cold with vomiting, and Spleen deficiency with diarrhea.

[Comments] Huang Lian, Huang Qin and Huang Bai are bitter and cold herbs; they all clear heat, dry dampness, drain fire and relieve toxicity. They are commonly combined for mutual reinforcement, named as San Huang, or three Huang.

# Huang Bai  *Phellodendron*

*Cortex Phellodendri*
*Bitter, cold; Kidney, Bladder, Large Intestine*

[Characteristics] With the same effects to dry dampness and relieve toxicity as Huang Lian, Huang Bai also descends downward, and is especially effective in eliminating damp-heat from the lower burner and draining *Xiang Huo*. It is often used to treat damp-heat jaundice, Damp-heat-type of Painful Urinary Dysfunction, excessive vaginal discharge, dysentery disorder, and Kidney yin insufficiency with deficient fire.

### FUNCTIONS • INDICATIONS & MAJOR COMBINATIONS

**1. Clear heat and dry dampness:**
- Patterns of damp-heat in the lower burner.
  - — Dysentery disorder. *+ Huang Lian, Bai Tou Weng*
  - — Jaundice. *+ Zhi Zi, Yin Chen Hao*
  - — Excessive turbid and yellow vaginal discharge. *+ Che Qian Zi*
  - — Heat-type of Painful Urinary Dysfunction. *+ Zhu Ye, Mu Tong*
  - — Red swollen painful feet and knees. *+ Cang Zhu, Niu Xi*

**2. Drain fire and relieve toxicity:**
- Excess heat and fire toxicity in the Triple Burner with high fever and irritability or sores and abscesses, etc. *+ Huang Lian, Zhi Zi*

**3. Eliminate deficient heat:**
- Kidney yin deficiency with ascending *Xiang Huo* inducing Steaming Bone Disorder, night sweating and nocturnal emission. *+ Zhi Mu*

[Dosage] 3-10 g. Fry with salt water may accelerate the herb to enter the Kidney channel and eliminate *Xiang Huo*.

[Precautions] Contraindicated in Spleen and Stomach deficient cold.

[Comments] ❶ According to the Physicians' Desk Reference published in China, the Chineses pinyin of Huang Bai is Huang Bo.

❷ Huang Bai is used to treat Steaming Bone Disorder, night sweating and nocturnal emission due to Kidney yin deficiency with ascending empty fire, known as *Xiang Huo*. It drains *Xiang Huo* and prevents fire to further injure the yin; it does not have any effect on nourishing the yin or tonifying the Kidney. Clinically, it is often combined with Zhi Mu.

# Long Dan Cao

*Radix Gentianae*
*Bitter, cold; Liver, Gallbladder, Stomach*

[Characteristics] Extremely bitter and cold in nature, Long Dan Cao is an herb that descends downward. It is especially effective in draining damp-heat from the Liver, Gallbladder and lower burner, as well as draining excess heat and constrained fire from the Liver and Gallbladder. It is appropriate for use in damp-heat jaundice, damp-heat in the lower burner, Liver fire blazing up with red swollen painful eyes, and extreme heat generating internal wind.

### FUNCTIONS • INDICATIONS & MAJOR COMBINATIONS

**1. Clear heat and dry dampness:**
- Damp-heat jaundice. *+ Yin Chen Hao, Zhi Zi*
- Damp-heat in the lower burner with external genital itchiness and rashes or excessive vaginal discharge. *+ Huang Bai, Ku Shen*

**2. Clear and drain excess Liver fire:**
- Liver fire blazing up with hypochondriac distention and pain, headache, red eyes and bitter taste in the mouth. *+ Chai Hu, Huang Qin*
- Extreme Liver fire generating internal wind with high fever, convulsions, and spasms in the extremities. *+ Gou Teng, Niu Huang*

[Dosage] 3-6 g.

[Precautions] Contraindicated in Spleen and Stomach deficient cold.

# Ku Shen $Sophora$

*Radix Sophorae Flavescentis*
*Bitter, cold; Heart, Liver, Stomach, Large Intestine, Bladder*

**[Characteristics]** Extremely bitter and cold, Ku Shen is an herb that descends downward; it specifically drains damp-heat from the lower burner. With similar effects as Huang Bai and Long Dan Cao, it is used for damp-heat in the lower burner; with similar effects as Huang Lian, it clears heat and alleviates dysentery. It can also disperse wind, kill parasites and stop itchiness.

**FUNCTIONS • INDICATIONS & MAJOR COMBINATIONS**

**1. Clear heat and dry dampness:**
- Patterns of damp-heat in the lower burner.
  - Diarrhea and dysentery disorders. *+ Mu Xiang*
  - Bloody stool and bleeding hemorrhoids. *+ Sheng Di Huang*
  - Jaundice. *+ Yin Chen Hao, Zhi Zi*
  - Thick yellow vaginal discharge. *+ Huang Bai, She Chuang Zi*

**2. Disperse wind, kill parasites and stop itchiness for skin itchiness due to damp toxins. Use as an external wash.**

**[Dosage]** 3-10 g.

**[Precautions]** Incompatible with Li Lu. Contraindicated in Spleen deficient cold.

# Qin Pi $Ash\ Bark$

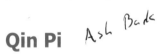

*Cortex Fraxini*
*Bitter, astringent, cold; Liver, Gallbladder, Large Intestine*

**[Characteristics]** Bitter, cold and astringent, Qin Pi clears and drains Liver fire to brighten the eyes. It also dries dampness and clears heat to alleviate dysentery.

**FUNCTIONS • INDICATIONS & MAJOR COMBINATIONS**

**1. Clear heat, dry dampness, relieve toxicity and alleviate dysentery:**
- Damp-heat or bloody dysentery. *+ Huang Lian, Bai Tou Weng*
- Damp-heat with excessive vaginal discharge. *+ Huang Bai*

**2. Clear the Liver and brighten the eyes:**
- Liver fire blazing up with red swollen painful eyes and formation of superficial visual obstruction. *+ Huang Lian, Jue Ming Zi*

**[Dosage]** 3-10 g.

Honeysuckle
flower

# Jin Yin Hua

*Flos Lonicerae*
*Sweet, cold; Lung, Stomach, Large Intestine*

[Characteristics] Cold to clear heat and relieve toxicity, aromatic to vent heat and disperse outward, it clears heat from the Heart and Stomach to relieve toxicity. It disperses wind-heat from the Lung channel to release the exterior. It can be used for heat toxicity with either sores or carbuncles, and all levels of Warm-Febrile Disease. Charred form can cool the blood and alleviate dysentery.

## FUNCTIONS • INDICATIONS & MAJOR COMBINATIONS

**1. Relieve toxicity and vent heat:**
- All levels of Warm-Febrile Disease.
  - — Protective level. *+ Lian Qiao, Bo He*
  - — Qi level. *+ Shi Gao, Zhi Mu*
  - — Nutritive and blood level. *+ Xi Jiao, Sheng Di Huang*

**2. Relieve toxicity and reduce swelling:**
- Heat toxicity with sores and abscesses. *+ Zi Hua Di Ding, Pu Gong Ying*
- Intestinal abscess with abdominal pain. *+ Da Huang, Mu Dan Pi*

**3. Cool the blood, relieve toxicity and alleviate dysentery for heat toxicity with bloody dysentery.**

[Dosage] 10-15 g. Small dose is recommended for exterior wind-heat condition; large dose is recommended for heat toxicity with sores and abscesses; charred form is used for heat toxicity with bloody dysentery.

[Comments] The alternative names are Yin Hua and Shuang Hua.

## [Addendum]
## Ren Dong Teng

*Caulis Lonicerae*

Also known as Yin Hua Teng, although having similar properties and effects as Jin Yin Hua, Ren Dong Teng has milder effect in relieving toxicity. Nevertheless, it eliminates wind, dampness and heat from the channels to alleviate pain for Wind-damp-heat Painful Obstruction with red, swollen and painful joints that are warm to touch and difficult to move. 10-20 g.

# Lian Qiao *Forsythia*

*Fructus Forsythiae*
*Bitter, slightly cold; Lung, Heart, Gallbladder*

**[Characteristics]** Light, ascending and floating to disperse, Lian Qiao disperses the exterior and vents the interior. It clears excess fire from the Heart channel, relieves toxicity and reduces swelling. It is used for exterior wind-heat, heat lodged in the nutritive level of Warm-Febrile Disease, and for pathogenic factors trapped in the Pericardium. It is effective in treating sores, carbuncles and swelling, and is regarded as the imperial herb for *Chuang Jia*.*

| FUNCTIONS • INDICATIONS & MAJOR COMBINATIONS |
|---|

**1. Relieve toxicity and vent heat:**
- Exterior wind-heat or the initial stage of Warm-Febrile Disease with fever, headache, slight thirst and sore throat. *+ Jin Yin Hua, Bo He*
- Heat lodged in the Pericardium with high fever, irritability and loss of consciousness. *+ Xi Jiao, Xuan Shen*

**2. Relieve toxicity, reduce abscess and dissipate nodules:**
- Heat toxicity with sores, abscesses, boils and swelling. *+ Jin Yin Hua, Ye Ju Hua*
- Scrofula. *+ Xia Ku Cao, Xuan Shen*

**[Dosage]** 6-15 g.

**[Comments]** *Chuang Jia*\*: First seen in <u>Shang Han Lun</u>, in which the author Zhang, Zhongjing referred *Chuang Jia* as those patients who suffer from chronic non-healing sores and ulcerations. According to the theory of "all patterns of pain, sores and ulcerations originate from the Heart", the presence of sores and ulcerations is related to Heart fire excess. Lian Qiao is especially effective in clearing excess heat from the Heart channel, relieving toxicity and reducing swelling; therefore, Lian Qiao is named as the imperial herb for *Chuang Jia*.

**Herbs that Clear Heat and Relieve Toxicity**

# *Indigo* *leaves* Da Qing Ye

*Folium Isatidis*
*Bitter, very cold; Heart, Lung, Stomach*

[Characteristics] Relieving toxicity, Da Qing Ye is especially effective in cooling the blood and reducing purpura and petechia. It enters both the qi level and blood level; it is often used for flaring fire in both qi and blood levels of Warm-Febrile Disease, and patterns of excess heat and fire toxicity.

**FUNCTIONS • INDICATIONS & MAJOR COMBINATIONS**

### 1. Cool the blood and reduce purpura and petechia:
- Flaring fire in both qi and blood levels of Warm-Febrile Disease with high fever, loss of consciousness, purpura and petechia or rashes, hematemesis, subcutaneous and mucosa hemorrhage. *+ Xi Jiao, Zhi Zi*

### 2. Clear heat and relieve toxicity:
- Excess heat and fire toxicity with swollen sore throat, sores in the mouth and tongue. *+ Xuan Shen, Shan Dou Gen*
- Toxic swelling, sores and carbuncles; topically apply the grounded fresh herb.
- Early stage of Warm-Febrile Disease. *+ Jin Yin Hua, Niu Bang Zi*

[Dosage] 10-15 g.

[Precautions] Contraindicated in Spleen and Stomach deficient cold.

[Addendum]
## Ban Lan Gen
### Radix Isatidis
Bitter and cold, it enters the Heart and Stomach channels. With similar effects as Da Qing Ye, Ban Lan Gen has stronger effects to cool the blood and relieve toxicity. It is often used for patterns of heat toxicity located around the head and face, such as facial erysipelas, mumps, swollen and sore throat, etc. Recently it is used to treat conditions such as influenza or hepatitis induced by viral infection. 10-15 g.

## Qing Dai
### Indigo Naturalis
Salty and cold, it enters the Liver, Lung and Stomach channels. With similar effects as Da Qing Ye, Qing Dai has stronger effect on clearing excess heat from the Liver channel. It is used for Liver fire generating internal wind or Liver fire invading the Lung with cough. 1.5-3 g. Take the powdered form with warm water.

# Pu Gong Ying *Dandelion*

*Herba Taraxaci*
*Bitter, sweet, cold; Liver, Stomach*

**[Characteristics]** Relieves toxicity, reduces abscesses and dissipates nodules. Pu Gong Ying is used for any pattern of heat toxicity with sores and abscesses. It is the primary herb for breast abscess.

**FUNCTIONS • INDICATIONS & MAJOR COMBINATIONS**

**1. Relieve toxicity and reduce abscess:**
- Breast abscess, use fresh form alone either by taking it orally or by applying the juice topically.
- Lung abscess. *+ Yu Xing Cao, Lu Gen*
- Intestinal abscess. *+ Da Huang, Mu Dan Pi*
- Heat toxicity with sores and abscesses. *+ Zi Hua Di Ding*

**2. Clear heat and drain dampness:**
- Damp-heat jaundice or Heat-type of Painful Urinary Dysfunction. *+ Yin Chen Hao, Jin Qian Cao*

**[Dosage]** 10-30 g. Double the dose when using fresh form.

# Zi Hua Di Ding *Viola, Tokyo violet*

*Herba Violae*
*Bitter, acrid, cold; Heart, Liver*

**[Characteristics]** With similar effects as Pu Gong Ying, Zi Hua Di Ding has a stronger effect in relieving toxicity. It is the primary herb for *Ding*\*.

**FUNCTIONS • INDICATIONS & MAJOR COMBINATIONS**

**Clear heat and relieve toxicity:**
- *Ding*, erysipelas and any pattern of heat toxicity with sores and abscesses, such as breast abscess, etc. *+ Pu Gong Ying, Jin Yin Hua*

**[Dosage]** 10-30 g. Double the dose when using fresh form.

**[Comments]** *Ding*\*: Is a severe suppurative pathological condition that occurs on the surface of the body with acute and critical onset. Despite the insignificant swelling, it is deeply rooted into the body like a nail, known and pronounced as *Ding* in Chinese. Therefore, this pathological condition is named *Ding*.

# Yu Xing Cao

*Herba Houttuyniae*
*Acrid, slightly cold; Lung*

[handwritten: Houttuynia]

[Characteristics] Clears heat, relieves toxicity and reduces abscess. Yu Xing Cao enters the Lung channel. It is the primary herb for Lung abscess. In addition, it clears heat and promotes urination.

**FUNCTIONS • INDICATIONS & MAJOR COMBINATIONS**

### 1. Relieve toxicity, reduce abscess, and promote purulent discharge:
- Lung abscess with coughing up thick yellow-green sputum or sputum mixed with purulent blood. *+ Jie Geng, Lu Gen*
- Lung heat with coughing up thick yellow sputum. *+ Huang Qin, Gua Lou*
- Heat toxicity with sores and abscesses. *+ Pu Gong Ying, Ye Ju Hua*

### 2. Used for Heat-type of Painful Urinary Dysfunction.

[Dosage] 10-30 g.


# Bai Jiang Cao

[handwritten: Patrinia]

*Herba cum Radice Patriniae*
*Acrid, bitter, slightly cold; Liver, Stomach, Large Intestine*

[Characteristics] Relieves toxicity, promotes purulent discharge, invigorates the blood and reduces abscess. Bai Jiang Cao is the primary herb for intestinal abscess. It also drains the constrained heat from the Lung.

**FUNCTIONS • INDICATIONS & MAJOR COMBINATIONS**

### 1. Relieve toxicity, reduce abscess, and promote purulent discharge:
- Intestinal abscess.
  — Unsuppurated. *+ Jin Yin Hua, Mu Dan Pi*
  — Suppurated. *+ Yi Yi Ren, Fu Zi*
- Lung abscess with coughing up thick yellow-green sputum or sputum mixed with purulent blood. *+ Yu Xing Cao, Pu Gong Ying*

### 2. Dispel blood stasis and alleviate pain for post-partum blood stasis with sharp pain in the lower abdomen.

[Dosage] 6-15 g.

# Ma Chi Xian

*purslane, portulaca*

*Herba Portulacae*
*Sour, cold; Liver, Large Intestine*

[Characteristics] Primarily entering the Large Intestine channel, it is used to treat Damp-heat-type of dysentery disorder. It also treats excessive vaginal discharge and Heat-type of Painful Urinary Dysfunction.

FUNCTIONS • INDICATIONS & MAJOR COMBINATIONS

**1. Relieve toxicity, cool the blood and alleviate dysentery:**
- Damp-heat dysentery disorder with diarrhea, purulent blood in the stool and tenesmus. *+ Huang Qin, Huang Lian*

**2. Used for excessive vaginal discharge, Heat-type or Blood-type of Painful Urinary Dysfunction.**

[Dosage] 30-60 g. Double the dosage when taken fresh form.


# Bai Tou Weng

*pulsatilla, Chinese anemone root*

*Radix Pulsatillae*
*Bitter, cold; Large Intestine*

[Characteristics] It is the primary herb for damp-heat dysentery disorder. Bai Tou Weng has a strong effect to cool the blood; it is especially effective for dysentery with blood in the stool.

FUNCTIONS • INDICATIONS & MAJOR COMBINATIONS

**1. Relieve toxicity, cool the blood and alleviate dysentery:**
- Damp-heat dysentery disorder with diarrhea, more blood than pus in the stool and tenesmus. *+ Huang Lian, Huang Bai*
- External genital itchiness or excessive vaginal discharge. Used as an external wash with the decoction. *+ Qin Pi, Ku Shen*

**2. Use for malarial disorder.** *+ Chai Hu, Huang Qin*

[Dosage] 6-15 g.

# Tu Fu Ling

*smooth greenbrier rhizome*

*Rhizoma Smilacis Glabrae*
*Sweet, bland, neutral; Liver, Stomach*

**[Characteristics]** Sweet and bland in nature, it drains dampness, clears heat as well as relieves toxicity.

**FUNCTIONS • INDICATIONS & MAJOR COMBINATIONS**

**Relieve toxicity and eliminate dampness:**
- Damp-heat causing abscesses, sores, furuncles and swelling. Mainly for topical application.
- Used for syphilis or mercury poisoning caused by the medication containing mercury for syphillis. *+ Jin Yin Hua, Bai Xian Pi*

**[Dosage]** 15-60 g.

# Bai Xian Pi

*cortex of Ch. dittany root*

*Cortex Dictamni*
*Bitter, cold; Spleen, Stomach*

**[Characteristics]** Relieves toxicity and eliminates dampness. It is often used in damp-heat sores and ulcerations with skin itchiness. It can also treat Damp-heat jaundice and Damp-heat Painful Obstruction.

**FUNCTIONS • INDICATIONS & MAJOR COMBINATIONS**

**1. Relieve toxicity, eliminate dampness and alleviate itchiness:**
- Damp-heat sores and ulcerations with purulent discharge or clammy and ulcerated skin with itchiness. *+ Ku Shen, Cang Zhu*

**2. Used for Damp-heat jaundice or Damp-heat Painful Obstruction.**

**[Dosage]** 6-10 g.

# She Gan

*Rhizoma Belamcandae*
*Bitter, cold; Lung*

**[Characteristics]** She Gan is especially effective in clearing phlegm-fire from the Lung to relieve toxicity and benefit the throat. It is often used for phlegm-fire blazing up that causes swollen sore throat.

**FUNCTIONS • INDICATIONS & MAJOR COMBINATIONS**

**1. Clear heat, relieve toxicity and benefit the throat:**
- Phlegm-fire blazing up with swollen sore throat. *+ Jie Geng, Gan Cao*

**2. Dispel phlegm and benefit the throat:**
- Excessive phlegm with coughing and wheezing.
  — Heat type. *+ Sang Bai Pi, Ma Dou Ling*
  — Cold type. *+ Ban Xia, Xi Xin*

**[Dosage]** 6-10 g.

**[Precautions]** Contraindicated during pregnancy.


# Shan Dou Gen

*bushy sophora*

*Radix Sophorae Tonkinensis*
*Bitter, cold; Lung*

**[Characteristics]** Extremely bitter and cold, it primarily enters the Lung channel. Shan Dou Gen clears and drains Lung heat and fire toxicity. It is the primary herb for swollen sore throat due to heat toxicity accumulation.

**FUNCTIONS • INDICATIONS & MAJOR COMBINATIONS**

**1. Relieve toxicity, reduce swelling and benefit the throat:**
- Heat toxicity accumulation with swollen sore throat.
  — Mild case. Gargle, swish and spit with the decoction of this herb alone.
  — Severe case. *+ Xuan Shen, She Gan*

**2. Damp-heat jaundice, toxic swelling, sores and carbuncles.**

**[Dosage]** 6-10 g.

**[Precautions]** Not recommended in Spleen and Stomach deficient cold.

**Herbs that Clear Heat and Relieve Toxicity**

# Chuan Xin Lian

*green chirette* (handwritten)

*Herba Andrographis*
*Bitter, cold; Lung, Stomach, Large Intestine, Small Intestine*

[Characteristics] It clears excess heat and fire toxicity from the Lung and Stomach, as well as eliminates damp-heat from the Large Intestine. It can be used for Lung heat cough, swollen sore throat, damp-heat dysentery or Damp-heat-type of Painful Urinary Dysfunction.

### FUNCTIONS • INDICATIONS & MAJOR COMBINATIONS

**1. Clear heat and relieve toxicity:**
   - Lung heat with coughing and wheezing. *+ Di Gu Pi, Sang Bai Pi*
   - Initial stage of Warm-Febrile Disease with fever and swollen sore throat. *+ Jin Yin Hua, Jie Geng*

**2. Clear heat and dry dampness:**
   - Damp-heat dysentery disorder. *+ Ma Chi Xian*
   - Damp-heat-type of Painful Urinary Dysfunction. *+ Che Qian Zi, Bai Mao Gen*

[Dosage] 6-15 g. Recently, it is often used in tablet, pill and powdered forms. Long-term usage or large dose could injure Stomach qi.

# Qing Hao *Sweet Wormwood*

*Herba Artemisiae Annuae*
*Bitter, acrid, cold; Liver, Gallbladder, Kidney*

**[Characteristics]** Bitter and cold in nature, it clears heat; aromatic in nature, it vents and disperses the lingering heat from the yin level. It is often used for warm and heat pathogenic factors that injure the yin with fever or Steaming Bone Disorder due to yin deficiency. It relieves summerheat and keeps malaria under control.

| FUNCTIONS • INDICATIONS & MAJOR COMBINATIONS |
| --- |
| **1. Reduce deficient heat:** <br> • Late stage of Warm-Febrile Disease, heat lingering in the yin level with fever at night that reduces in the morning, absence of sweating as fever reduces, and post Warm-Febrile Disease with unremitting low grade temperature. *+ Bie Jia, Mu Dan Pi* <br> • Yin deficiency with heat, such as low grade fever or Steaming Bone Disorder. *+ Qin Jiao, Zhi Mu* |
| **2. Relieve summerheat:** <br> • Exterior summerheat with fever, irritability, sweating and thirst. *+ Lian Qiao, Hua Shi* |
| **3. Keep malaria under control and relieve heat:** <br> • Malarial disorder with alternating fever and chills, especially appropriate if it is accompanied by summerheat-dampness. *+ Huang Qin, Ban Xia* |

**[Dosage]** 3-10 g. Not recommended to decoct for long periods of time.

**Herbs that Eliminate Deficient Heat**

# Bai Wei

*Radix Cynanchi Atrati*
*Bitter, salty, cold; Liver, Stomach*

**[Characteristics]** It clears heat and cools the blood. Bai Wei clears excess heat and reduces deficient heat, as well as promotes urination.

### FUNCTIONS • INDICATIONS & MAJOR COMBINATIONS

**1. Clear heat and cool the blood:**
- Heat lodged in the blood level of Warm-Febrile Disease with high fever. *+ Xi Jiao, Xuan Shen*
- Yin deficiency with fever or Steaming Bone Disorder. *+ Di Gu Pi*

**2. Promote urination and unblock the obstruction in the urinary tract:**
- Heat-type or Blood-type of Painful Urinary Dysfunction. *+ Hua Shi, Mu Tong*

**3. Used for heat toxicity with sores and abscesses or swollen sore throat.**

**[Dosage]** 3-10 g.

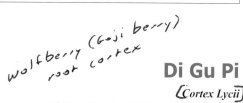

wolfberry (Goji berry)
root cortex

# Di Gu Pi

*Cortex Lycii*
*Bitter, bland, cold; Lung, Liver, Kidney*

**[Characteristics]** Sweet and cold in nature, it clears heat and moistens dryness. Di Gu Pi is the primary herb for yin deficiency with fever or Steaming Bone Disorder. It can also clear and drain Lung heat.

### FUNCTIONS • INDICATIONS & MAJOR COMBINATIONS

**1. Cool the blood and reduce deficient heat:**
- Yin deficiency with fever, childhood *Gan Re* and Steaming Bone Disorder. *+ Zhi Mu, Bie Jia*
- Wasting and Thirsting Disorder. *+ Tian Hua Fen, Sheng Di Huang*
- Heat causing the blood to move recklessly with hematemesis, subcutaneous and mucosa hemorrhage. *+ Bai Mao Gen, Ce Bai Ye*

**2. Clear and drain Lung heat:**
- Lung heat with coughing and wheezing. *+ Sang Bai Pi, Gan Cao*

**[Dosage]** 6-15 g.

---

**Herbs that Eliminate Deficient Heat**

# Yin Chai Hu

*Radix Stellariae*
*Sweet, slightly cold; Liver, Stomach*

[Characteristics] With the same effect of reducing deficient heat as Di Gu Pi, Yin Chai Hu also clears *Gan Re*\*. It is the primary herb for *Gan Re* in childhood.

| FUNCTIONS • INDICATIONS & MAJOR COMBINATIONS |
|---|
| **1. Reduce deficient heat:**<br>• Yin deficiency with fever and night sweating. *+ Di Gu Pi, Bie Jia* |
| **2. Clear *Gan Re*:**<br>• *Gan Re* in childhood with emaciation, abdominal distention, sallow complexion and red eyes. *+ Zhi Zi, Huang Qin* |

[Dosage] 3-10 g.

[Comments] *Gan Re*\*: Refers to the condition of deficient heat with emaciation, sallow complexion, thin hair, and exhaustion of fluid due to chronic nutritional impairment and heat accumulation in childhood.


# Hu Huang Lian

*Rhizoma Picrorhizae*
*Bitter, cold; Heart, Liver, Stomach, Large Intestine*

[Characteristics] It has similar effects to reduce deficient heat and clear *Gan Re* as Yin Chai Hu; moreover, Hu Huang Lian is bitter and cold in nature to eliminate damp-heat. It is used to treat damp-heat dysentery disorder with similar effect as Huang Lian.

| FUNCTIONS • INDICATIONS & MAJOR COMBINATIONS |
|---|
| **1. Reduce deficient heat:**<br>• Yin deficiency with fever and night sweating. *+ Yin Chai Hu* |
| **2. Clear *Gan Re*:**<br>• *Gan Re* in childhood. *+ Bai Zhu, Shi Jun Zi* |
| **3. Eliminate damp-heat:**<br>• Damp-heat diarrhea and dysentery, swollen and painful hemorrhoid. Apply topically or take orally. |

[Dosage] 3-10 g.

**Herbs that Eliminate Deficient Heat**

## [Remarks & Differentiations]

### Shi Gao — Zhi Mu

|   | Shi Gao | Zhi Mu |
|---|---------|--------|
| **C** | Drain fire from the Lung and Stomach. Clear excess heat in either qi level or yang brightness stage. | |
| **D** | • Applied in excess heat only.<br><br>• Calcined to generate tissue. | • Nourishes yin of the Lung, Stomach and Kidney; applied in either excess or deficient heat.<br>• Enters the Kidney to drain *Xiang Huo*. |

### Lu Gen — Zhu Ye

|   | Lu Gen | Zhu Ye |
|---|--------|--------|
| **C** | Clear heat, generate fluid and promote urination. | |
| **D** | • Mainly enters the Lung channel to clear heat and transform phlegm.<br>• Enters the Stomach to clear heat and stop vomiting. | • Mainly enters the Heart channel to clear heat and eliminate irritability. |

### Xia Ku Cao — Jue Ming Zi

|   | Xia Ku Cao | Jue Ming Zi |
|---|-----------|-------------|
| **C** | Clear heat from the Liver and brighten the eyes. | |
| **D** | • Clears heat and dissipates nodules for goiter and scrofula. | • Moistens the intestines and unblocks the obstruction of bowel movements. |

### Xi Jiao — Sheng Di Huang

|   | Xi Jiao | Sheng Di Huang |
|---|---------|----------------|
| **C** | Clear heat and cool the blood, combined for mutual reinforcement. | |
| **D** | • Strongly relieves heat toxicity, clears heat from the Heart and calms convulsions. | • Sweet, cold, moist and juicy to strongly nourish the yin for patterns of yin deficiency. |

## Sheng Di Huang — Xuan Shen — Mu Dan Pi

|   | Sheng Di Huang | Xuan Shen | Mu Dan Pi |
|---|---|---|---|
| C | Clear heat and cool the blood. For heat lodged in the nutritive and blood level of Warm-Febrile Disease. | | |
| D | • Sweet, cold, moist and juicy to nourish the yin for patterns of yin deficiency. | • Salty and cold to soften hardness, relieve toxicity, and dissipate nodules for scrofula and sores due to heat toxicity. | • Also invigorate the blood and dispel stasis for blood stasis due to heat consuming fluid in the blood. |

## Huang Qin — Huang Lian — Huang Bai

|   | Huang Qin | Huang Lian | Huang Bai |
|---|---|---|---|
| C | Clear heat, dry dampness, drain fire and relieve toxicity. Commonly combined for mutual reinforcement, known as San Huang. | | |
| D | • Primarily clears heat from the Lung. <br> • Clears heat and calms the fetus. | • Mainly drains fire from the Heart and Stomach. <br> • Clears damp-heat from the Stomach and intestines. | • Enters the Kidney to drain *Xiang Huo*. <br> • Clears damp-heat from the lower burner. |

## Huang Bai — Long Dan Cao

|   | Huang Bai | Long Dan Cao |
|---|---|---|
| C | Effectively drain damp-heat from the lower burner. | |
| D | • Enters the Kidney to drain *Xiang Huo*. | • Enters the Liver and Gallbladder to drain excess heat and constrained fire. |

## Jin Yin Hua — Lian Qiao

|   | Jin Yin Hua | Lian Qiao |
|---|---|---|
| C | Relieve toxicity, vent heat and reduce swelling. For Warm-Febrile Disease and toxic sores, carbuncles and swelling. | |
| D | • Powerfully disperses wind-heat. <br> • Charred to cool the blood and alleviate dysentery. | • Clears excess fire from the Heart. <br> • Relieves toxicity and reduces swelling, the impeiral herb for *Chuang Jia*. |

**Herbs that Clear Heat**

## Pu Gong Ying — Zi Hua Di Ding

|   | **Pu Gong Ying** | **Zi Hua Di Ding** |
|---|---|---|
| **C** | Relieve toxicity and reduce abscesses. Combined for mutual reinforcement for toxic sores and carbuncles. | |
| **D** | • The primary herb for breast abscess. | • Effectively relieves toxicity, the primary herb for *Ding*. |

## Yu Xing Cao — Bai Jiang Cao

|   | **Yu Xing Cao** | **Bai Jiang Cao** |
|---|---|---|
| **C** | Relieve toxicity and promote purulent discharge. | |
| **D** | • Primarily for Lung abscess. | • Primarily for intestinal abscess. |

## She Gan — Shan Dou Gen

|   | **She Gan** | **Shan Dou Gen** |
|---|---|---|
| **C** | Relieve toxicity and benefit the throat for swollen sore throat. | |
| **D** | • Relieves toxicity and clears phlegm-heat for phlegm-fire blazing up causing swollen sore throat. | • Extremely bitter and cold, treats heat toxicity accumulation causing swollen sore throat. |

## Qin Pi — Ma Chi Xian — Bai Tou Weng

|   | **Qin Pi** | **Ma Chi Xian** | **Bai Tou Weng** |
|---|---|---|---|
| **C** | Dry dampness and relieve toxicity for damp-heat dysentery disorder. | | |
| **D** | • Can also clear the Liver and brighten the eyes. | • Also treats excessive vaginal discharge and Painful Urinary Dysfunction. | • Has the strongest effect to relieve toxicity, cool the blood, and is the primary herb for dysentery. |

## Qing Hao — Di Gu Pi — Yin Chai Hu

|   | **Qing Hao** | **Di Gu Pi** | **Yin Chai Hu** |
|---|---|---|---|
| **C** | Reduce deficient heat for yin deficiency with heat. | | |
| **D** | • Relieves summerheat. | • Drains Lung heat. | • Clears *Gan Re*. |

**Huang Lian — Hu Huang Lian**

|   | Huang Lian | Hu Huang Lian |
|---|---|---|
| **C** | Bitter and cold to clear heat and dry dampness. For damp-heat dysentery disorder. ||
| **D** | • Drains excess fire from the Heart and Stomach. | • Reduces deficient heat for yin deficiency with heat.<br>• Clears *Gan Re*. |

# HERBS THAT

## Drain Downward 3

Accelerating peristalsis or lubricating the intestines to facilitate bowel movements is the primary function of herbs in this category.

The majority of these herbs are bitter, cold and descending to unblock the obstruction of bowel movements and guide out accumulations, force out congested fluids and reduce edema. Some herbs eliminate accumulations and excess heat in the Stomach and intestines by way of bowel movements. Herbs in this category are also used to treat fecal impaction, constipation, edema with fullness and distention.

Herbs that drain downward are further subcategorized into the following: (1) purgatives, (2) moist laxatives, and (3) harsh expellants. The moist laxatives are gentler in action whereas, the other two groups are more aggressive because they tend to injure the righteous qi; therefore they should be used with caution.

It is recommended to discontinue the use of these herbs once the therapeutic effects are achieved. Due to their toxic and aggressive effects, refer to the dosage, methods of application, process and precautions for further details.

# Da Huang

*Radix et Rhizoma Rhei*
*Bitter, cold; Spleen, Stomach, Large Intestine, Liver, Heart*

[Characteristics] Bitter and cold, it purges heat; Da Huang has a strong purgative effect and it descends downward. It mainly enters the Stomach and Large Intestine to eliminate accumulations, excess heat and fire toxicity by promoting bowel movements. It is the primary herb for Yang Brightness Organ Stage Disorder and heat accumulation with fecal impaction. It also enters the Heart and Liver, or the blood level, to cool the blood and relieve toxicity, invigorate the blood and transform blood stasis. It is used for patterns of heat toxicity with sores and carbuncles, heat causing the blood to move recklessly with bleeding, and blood stasis. It also clears and eliminates damp-heat to treat jaundice and Painful Urinary Dysfunction.

**FUNCTIONS • INDICATIONS & MAJOR COMBINATIONS**

### 1. Purge heat and accumulations:
- Yang Brightness Organ Stage Disorder with high fever, delirium, fecal impaction, focal distention and abdominal pain. *+ Mang Xiao*
- Cold accumulation with constipation. *+ Fu Zi, Gan Jiang*
- Excessive heat injuring yin with constipation. *+ Xuan Shen*
- Damp-heat dysentery with blood in the stool. *+ Mu Xiang, Bing Lang*

### 2. Cool the blood and relieve toxicity:
- Heat causing the blood to move recklessly with hematemesis, subcutaneous and mucosa hemorrhaging. *+ Huang Qin, Huang Lian*
- Upward attacks of excess heat and fire toxicity with swollen sore throat, red eyes, sores and abscesses. *+ Zhi Zi, Jin Yin Hua*
- Intestinal abscess. *+ Tao Ren, Mu Dan Pi*

### 3. Invigorate the blood and transform blood stasis:
- Blood stasis with amenorrhea, post-partum lochioschesis and abdominal pain. *+ Tao Ren*
- Traumatic blood stasis. *+ Ru Xiang, Tao Ren*

### 4. Clear heat and drain dampness:
- Damp-heat jaundice. *+ Yin Chen Hao, Zhi Zi*
- Heat-type of Painful Urinary Dysfunction. *+ Che Qian Zi, Mu Tong*

[Dosage] 3-10 g. Using raw herb or adding it near the end to get a stronger purgative effect; decocted for long time will lessen the effect. Wine-fried form can strengthen its effect to invigorate the blood; charred is used to stop bleeding.

[Precautions] Contraindicated in pregnancy, menstruation and breastfeeding.

# Mang Xiao

*Natrii Sulfas*
*Salty, bitter, cold; Stomach, Large Intestine*

[Characteristics] With similar yet milder properties and effects than Da Huang, Mang Xiao is a salty and cold herb that softens hardness and moistens dryness. It is the primary herb to treat dry fecal impaction due to excess heat. Topically it is used to clear heat and reduce swelling.

| FUNCTIONS • INDICATIONS & MAJOR COMBINATIONS |
| --- |
| **1. Purge fire, soften hardness and moisten dryness:** <br> • Yang Brightness Organ Stage Disorder. *+ Da Huang, Zhi Shi* |
| **2. For fire toxicity with sore throat, sores in the mouth, red eyes and breast abscess, apply topically.** |

[Dosage] 6-15 g. Dissolve in strained decoction.

[Precautions] Contraindicated during pregnancy.

[Comments] According to various processes, there are three types of Mang Xiao:

**Pu Xiao**, containing more sediments, is often applied topically.

**Mang Xiao**, relatively pure, can be taken orally.

**Xuan Ming Fen**, the purest, or the dehydrated form, is applied topically in oral cavity or for ophthalmologic conditions.


# Fan Xie Ye

*Folium Sennae*
*Sweet, bitter, cold; Large Intestine*

[Characteristics] Having a moist consistency to lubricate the intestines, Fan Xie Ye is used as a mild laxative at a small dose; at higher dose, it has a stronger purgative effect, similar to Da Huang, to purge heat accumulation.

| FUNCTIONS • INDICATIONS & MAJOR COMBINATIONS |
| --- |
| **Purge heat and guide out the accumulations:** <br> • Heat accumulation with constipation. *+ Zhi Shi, Hou Po* |

[Dosage] 1.5-3 g. for a mild laxative effect; 5-10 g. for a purgative effect. Soak in hot water to make tea.

[Precautions] Contraindicated in pregnancy, breastfeeding and menstruation.

**Purgatives**

# Huo Ma Ren

*Fructus Cannabis*
*Sweet, neutral; Spleen, Large Intestine*

**[Characteristics]** Sweet, neutral and moist consistency, Huo Ma Ren contains rich oil. It is extremely effective in moistening the intestines and unblocking the obstruction of bowel movements. It can also tonify and nourish the deficiency. It is suitable for constipation in chronic illnesses, general weakness, post-partum, and the elderly with blood deficiency, lack of the fluid and intestinal dryness.

**FUNCTIONS • INDICATIONS & MAJOR COMBINATIONS**

**Moisten the intestines and unblock the obstruction of bowel movements:**
- Constipation in those with general weakness, and in the elderly with blood deficiency, lack of the fluid and intestinal dryness.
  *+ Dang Gui, Shu Di Huang*

**[Dosage]** 10-30 g.
**[Comments]** The alternative name is Ma Zi Ren.

# Yu Li Ren

*Semen Pruni*
*Acrid, bitter, sweet, neutral; Spleen, Large Intestine, Small Intestine*

**[Characteristics]** It has the same effects as Huo Ma Ren to moisten the intestines and unblock the obstruction of bowel movements; however, Yu Li Ren does not nourish nor tonify. Therefore, it is indicated for excess conditions, and is used with caution in deficiency. It also promotes urination.

**FUNCTIONS • INDICATIONS & MAJOR COMBINATIONS**

**1. Moisten the intestines and unblock the obstruction of bowel movements:**
- Intestinal dryness with constipation. *+ Huo Ma Ren*

**2. Promote urination and reduce edema:**
- Edema with abdominal distention. *+ Sang Bai Pi, Chi Xiao Dou*

**[Dosage]** 3-10 g.

# Gan Sui

*Radix Kansui*
*Bitter, sweet, cold, toxic; Lung, Kidney, Large Intestine*

[Characteristics] It induces severe watery diarrhea and promotes urination. Gan Sui eliminates the pathogenic water through bowel movements and urinations. It is an extreme harsh expellant that can drain excessive water and force out congested fluids; therefore, it can only be used in excess conditions of edema with distention and fullness. Topical application of the raw herb can reduce swelling, relieve toxicity and treat sores and carbuncles.

| FUNCTIONS • INDICATIONS & MAJOR COMBINATIONS |
|---|
| **1. Drain water and force out congested fluids:** <br> • Excess conditions of either edema or fluids accumulation in the abdominal cavity. *+ Da Ji, Da Zao* |
| **2. Reduce swelling and relieve toxicity:** <br> • Heat toxicity with sores and carbuncles, often use topical application. |

[Dosage] 0.5-1 g. Should be added to pill or made into powdered form. Fry with vinegar to reduce toxicity; raw form for topical application only.

[Precautions] Incompatible with Gan Cao. Contraindicated during pregnancy.


# Da Ji

*Radix Euphorbiae Pekinensis*
*Bitter, acrid, cold, toxic; Lung, Kidney, Large Intestine*

[Characteristics] Similar to but has milder effects compared to Gan Sui.

| FUNCTIONS • INDICATIONS & MAJOR COMBINATIONS |
|---|
| **1. Drain water and force out congested fluids:** <br> • Excess conditions of either edema or fluids accumulation in the abdominal cavity. *+ Gan Sui, Da Zao* |
| **2. Reduce swelling and relieve toxicity:** <br> • Heat toxicity with sores and carbuncles, often use topical application. |

[Dosage] 1.5-3 g. Use 1 g. in powdered form. Vinegar-fried to reduce toxicity.

[Precautions] Incompatible with Gan Cao. Contraindicated during pregnancy.

**Harsh Expellants**

# Yuan Hua

*Flos Genkwa*
*Acrid, bitter, cold, toxic; Lung, Kidney, Large Intestine*

[Characteristics] Yuan Hua is extremely effective in draining and expelling out congested fluids from the upper body or chest and hypochondriac regions. It kills parasites and treats sores when applied topically.

### FUNCTIONS • INDICATIONS & MAJOR COMBINATIONS

**1. Drain water and force out congested fluids:**
- Systemic and facial edema, congested fluids in the chest or hypochondriac region. *+ Gan Sui*

**2. Kill parasites and treat ringworms:**
- Infestation of stubborn ringworms on the body or on the head. Use powdered form for topical application.

[Dosage] 1.5-3 g. Use 0.6 g. in powdered form; vinegar-fried to reduce toxicity.

[Precautions] Incompatible with Gan Cao. Contraindicated during pregnancy.

# Qian Niu Zi

*Semen Pharbitidis*
*Bitter, cold, toxic; Lung, Kidney, Large Intestine*

[Characteristics] Less effective in forcing out congested fluids compared with Gan Sui, Da Ji and Yuan Hua; however, Qian Niu Zi can direct qi downward and eliminate accumulations.

### FUNCTIONS • INDICATIONS & MAJOR COMBINATIONS

**1. Force out congested fluids:**
- Excess condition of edema with distention and fullness. *+ Gan Sui*

**2. Damp-heat accumulation with constipation.**

**3. Intestinal parasites with abdominal pain.**

[Dosage] 3-10 g. crush for decoction. Use 1.5-3 g. in powdered form. Frying will moderate the aggressive effects.

[Precautions] Contraindicated during pregnancy.

[Comments] The alternative names are Hei Bai Chou and Er Chou.

# Ba Dou

*Fructus Crotonis*
*Acrid, hot, extremely toxic; Lung, Stomach, Large Intestine*

[Characteristics] Acrid and hot, Ba Dou is an extremely toxic herb for forcing out cold accumulation. This important harsh expellant is primarily used for condition of cold type food stagnation with abdominal distention and pain, and fecal impaction. It also can expel phlegm, benefit the throat and promote purulent discharge.

### FUNCTIONS • INDICATIONS & MAJOR COMBINATIONS

**1. Force out cold accumulation:**
- Critical condition of cold type of food stagnation obstructing the intestines with abdominal distention and pain, and fecal impaction. *+ Gan Jiang, Da Huang*
- Severe case of childhood food stagnation with excessive sputum and convulsions. Use Ba Dou Shuang *+ Shen Qu*

**2. Drain water and reduce edema:**
- Excess type of ascites and edema. *+ Xing Ren*
- Late stage of schistosomiasis with cirrhosis and ascites. *+ Cang Zhu, Chen Pi*

**3. Expel phlegm and benefit the throat:**
- Obstructive pharyngolaryngeal inflammation with excessive sputum, tachypnea, and stifling sensation in the chest and diaphragm. Spray Ba Dou Shuang into the throat.

**4. Apply topically to promote perforation of the suppurated abscesses.**

[Dosage] To reduce toxicity for clinical application, this herb is often processed into the defatty form, called Ba Dou Shuang. 0.1-0.3 g. Add to pills for oral administration.

[Precautions] Antagonized with Qian Niu Zi. Contraindicated during pregnancy or in those with general weakness. Avoid taking this herb together with hot beverages to prevent aggravation of purgative effects.

### Da Huang — Mang Xiao

|   | Da Huang | Mang Xiao |
|---|----------|-----------|
| C | Drain heat and unblock the obstruction of bowel movements. Combined for mutual reinforcement in excess heat accumulation with impaction. Apply topically for painful swelling, sores and carbuncles. | |
| D | • Strong purgative effect, descends to drain fire, cool the blood, and relieve toxicity.<br>• Invigorates the blood and expels stasis.<br>• Clears and drains damp-heat. | • Salty and cold in nature to soften hardness and moisten dryness. |

### Huo Ma Ren — Yu Li Ren

|   | Huo Ma Ren | Yu Li Ren |
|---|-----------|-----------|
| C | Moisten the intestines and unblock the obstruction of bowel movements. Combined for mutual reinforcement to treat constipation due to dryness. | |
| D | • With tonifying and nourishing effect for deficient conditions. | • Works well in excess conditions with lack of tonification function.<br>• Promotes urination and reduces edema. |

### Da Huang — Ba Dou

|   | Da Huang | Ba Dou |
|---|----------|--------|
| C | Force out the accumulations as harsh expellants. | |
| D | • Bitter and cold for heat accumulation and impaction. | • Acrid, hot, extremely toxic, forces out the cold accumulation for cold type of food stagnation.<br>• Drains water and reduces edema. |

# HERBS THAT

## Dispel Wind-Dampness 4

Expelling wind-dampness and unblocking painful obstructions are the main functions of herbs in this category. In general, they are acrid and bitter, dispersing and drying in nature to eliminate wind-dampness from the exterior, from the joints, muscles, meridians and collaterals. However, some herbs also relax the sinews, unblock obstructions in the collaterals to relieve pain, and tonify the Liver and Kidney to benefit the sinews and bones. Wind-dampness Painful Obstruction, spasms and contractions of the sinews, numbness of the limbs, soreness and weakness of the extremities are some conditions that can be treated with herbs that expel wind-dampness.

Based on various pathologies, select the appropriate herbs accordingly. Herbs that dispel wind-dampness are normally combined with herbs that expel wind, herbs that disperse cold, herbs that clear heat, and herbs that tonify the Liver and Kidney to benefit the sinews and bones.

The pathogenesis of Painful Obstruction is usually chronic and requires long-term therapy. For long-term use and easy administration, these herbs are often prepared in tincture, pill or powdered forms. The former is prepared with ethanol to enhance its strength.

*1° for β. Syndrome*

# Du Huo

*Radix Angelicae Pubescentis*
*Acrid, bitter, warm; Liver, Kidney, Bladder*

**[Characteristics]** Acrid to disperse, warm to unblock the obstruction, bitter and drying to eliminate the dampness, Du Huo tends to act on the interior and lower half of the body. It effectively dispels wind-cold-damp in the lower half of the body to unblock the obstruction and alleviate pain; it is also used to treat Lesser Yin headache radiating to the teeth and cheeks. Because of its gentle therapeutic effects, it is generally used for chronic pain.

| FUNCTIONS • INDICATIONS & MAJOR COMBINATIONS |
|---|
| **1. Dispel wind-dampness and alleviate pain:** *Yao Yao* <br> • Wind-cold-damp Painful Obstruction with pain in the joints and limbs, especially effective for those of the lower half of the body. <br> *+ Du Zhong, Sang Ji Sheng* |
| **2. Release the exterior and disperse cold:** <br> • Exterior wind-cold accompanied by dampness with pain and heaviness of the head and body. *+ Qiang Huo, Fang Feng* <br> • Lesser Yin headache with pain radiating to the teeth and cheeks. *+ Xi Xin, Chuan Xiong* |

**[Dosage]** 3-10 g.

**[Comments]** Du Huo and Qiang Huo have similar natures and functions. Both dispel wind, disperse cold, eliminate dampness and alleviate pain; therefore, these two herbs are usually combined together to treat Wind-cold-damp Painful Obstruction. Qiang Huo tends to act on the exterior and the upper half of the body. It primarily treats the exterior conditions of wind-cold with dampness, and Wind-cold-damp Painful Obstruction affecting the upper half of the body; Qiang Huo is the guiding herb that dispels wind for Greater Yang channels. Du Huo, on the contrary, tends to act on the interior and lower half of the body. It is mainly used for Wind-cold-damp Painful Obstruction affecting the lower half of the body; Du Huo is the guiding herb that dispels wind for Lesser Yin channels. The combination of these two herbs, known as Er Huo, or two Huo, is used to treat painful obstruction affecting the entire body.

*Also Shaoyin HA 2°*

---

# Wei Ling Xian

*Radix Clematidis*
*Acrid, salty, warm; Bladder*

**[Characteristics]** Wei Ling Xian is recognized by its powerful migrating ability. It travels into all twelve channels; therefore, it is an important herb for all conditions related to Wind-dampness Painful Obstruction, regardless of where the locations. It also softens the fish bones lodged in the throat.

| FUNCTIONS • INDICATIONS & MAJOR COMBINATIONS |
|---|
| **1. Disperse wind-damp, unblock obstruction and alleviate pain:**<br>  • Wind-dampness Painful Obstruction with painful joints and numb limbs. *+ Fang Feng, Chuan Xiong* |
| **2. For fish bones lodged in the throat, slowly sip the decoction.** |

**[Dosage]** 6-10 g. May use up to 30 g. to soften the fish bones.

**[Precautions]** Not recommended for long-term use.

# Mu Gua

*Fructus Chaenomelis*
*Sour, slightly warm; Liver, Spleen*

**[Characteristics]** With the sour, warm and aromatic properties, Mu Gua relaxes the sinews and invigorates the circulation in the collaterals, transforms dampness and harmonizes the Stomach. It is primarily used for Wind-dampness Painful Obstruction, especially effective for spasms of the sinews. It is also used for severe vomiting and diarrhea with muscular spasms.

| FUNCTIONS • INDICATIONS & MAJOR COMBINATIONS |
|---|
| **1. Relax the sinews and invigorate the circulation in the collaterals:**<br>  • Painful obstruction with muscle cramps. *+ Ru Xiang, Mo Yao* |
| **2. Transform dampness and harmonize the Stomach:**<br>  • Dampness accumulating in the middle causing severe vomiting and diarrhea with muscle cramps of the calves. *+ Wu Zhu Yu, Huang Lian*<br>  • Indigestion. *+ Shan Zha, Shen Qu* |
| **3. It also generates the fluid and is used for insufficiency of Stomach fluid.** |

**[Dosage]** 6-10 g. Use the tincture form to treat painful obstruction.

**Herbs that Dispel Wind-Dampness**

# Hai Feng Teng

*Caulis Piperis Kadsurae*
*Acrid, bitter, slightly warm; Liver*

**[Characteristics]** Acrid, bitter and slightly warm, it is often used for painful obstruction with the absence of heat signs. Hai Feng Teng has strong effects of dispersing and invigorating.

---
**FUNCTIONS • INDICATIONS & MAJOR COMBINATIONS**

**Dispel wind-dampness and unblock the channels:**
- Wind-dampness Painful Obstruction with spasms of the sinews, and traumatic injuries with body ache. *+ Du Huo, Qin Jiao*

---

**[Dosage]** 6-15 g.

# Bai Hua She

*Agkistrodon*
*Sweet, salty, warm, toxic; Liver*

**[Characteristics]** Being sweet and salty, it enters the Liver channel, or the blood level. It penetrates deeply into the bones to search and gather the wind trapped within, and it invigorates the circulation in the collaterals to quiet the convulsions; Bai Hua She treats all patterns of external wind invading or internal wind swirling.

---
**FUNCTIONS • INDICATIONS & MAJOR COMBINATIONS**

**1. Dispel wind and unblock the channels:**
- Stubborn Wind-dampness Painful Obstruction. *+ Du Huo, Dang Gui*
- Hemiplegia secondary to wind stroke. *+ Huang Qi, Dang Gui*

**2. Extinguish wind and quiet the convulsion:**
- Tetanus and opisthotonos. *+ Quan Xie, Tian Ma*
- Childhood convulsion due to high fever. *+ Dan Nan Xing*

---

**[Dosage]** 3-10 g. 1-1.5 g. when using the powdered form.

**[Addendum]**
## Wu Shao She
### Zaocys Dhumnades
Sweet, neutral and non-toxic, it has similar effects to but milder than Bai Hua She.
6-10 g. 2-3 g. when using the powdered form.

# Qin Jiao

*Radix Gentianae Macrophyllae*
*Bitter, acrid, slightly cold; Liver, Gallbladder, Stomach*

[Characteristics] Acrid to disperse wind, bitter to dry dampness, it is especially effective in dispelling wind-dampness and relaxing the sinews. Recognizing that "herbs expelling wind are drying", Qin Jiao is an exception because it is relatively soft and moist. This herb is used in conditions of Wind-dampness Painful Obstruction with muscle spasms regardless of acute or chronic onset, cold or heat patterns. With slightly cold nature, it is more effective in treating Heat-type of Painful Obstruction. Qin Jiao also clears deficient heat, eliminates *Gan Re* and jaundice.

FUNCTIONS • INDICATIONS & MAJOR COMBINATIONS

### 1. Dispel wind-dampness, relax the sinews and unblock the collaterals:
- Wind-dampness Painful Obstruction with spasms of the sinews and difficult movement of the extremities.
  — Conditions prone to heat. *+ Ren Dong Teng, Fang Ji*
  — Conditions prone to cold. *+ Qiang Huo, Du Huo*
- Hemiplegia secondary to wind stroke with spasms and contractures of the extremities. *+ Dang Gui, Bai Shao*

### 2. Clear deficient heat:
- Yin deficiency with Steaming Bone Disorder and tidal fever. *+ Qing Hao, Bie Jia*
- Childhood *Gan Re*. *+ Shi Jun Zi, Bing Lang*

### 3. Clear heat, drain dampness and eliminate jaundice:
- Damp-heat jaundice. *+ Yin Chen Hao, Zhi Zi*

[Dosage] 6-10 g.

# Fang Ji

*Radix Stephaniae Tetrandrae*
*Bitter, acrid, cold; Bladder, Kidney, Spleen*

[Characteristics] Acrid and dispersing, it dispels wind; bitter and descending, it promotes urination; cold in nature, it clears heat; therefore, Fang Ji dispels wind, drains damp-heat, unblocks the channels and alleviates pain. It is very effective for the treatment of Damp-heat Painful Obstruction. It also can promote urination to reduce swelling; therefore, it is the primary herb for *Feng Shui** or *Pi Shui**.

### FUNCTIONS • INDICATIONS & MAJOR COMBINATIONS

**1. Dispel wind-dampness and unblock the painful obstruction:**
- Damp-heat Painful Obstruction with red swollen painful joints that are warm to touch. *+ Yi Yi Ren, Hua Shi*
- Wind-cold-damp Painful Obstruction. *+ Fu Zi, Fang Feng*

**2. Promote urination and reduce swelling:**
- *Feng Shui* with edema of the head and face. *+ Huang Qi, Bai Zhu*
- *Pi Shui* with systemic edema. *+ Huang Qi, Gui Zhi*
- Damp-heat accumulation with abdominal distention and edema. *+ Ting Li Zi, Da Huang*

[Dosage] 6-10 g.

[Comments] ❶ There are two different species of Fang Ji:

**Han Fang Ji**, with good effects in draining dampness and reducing swelling, is often used for conditions of edema.

**Mu Fang Ji**, with good effects in dispersing wind and alleviating pain, is often used for Wind-dampness Painful Obstruction.

❷ *Feng Shui**: Is a type of edema due to impaired function of water metabolism, caused by exterior-contracted wind and impaired function of Lung qi to disperse and descend. Manifestations are acute onset, and include aversion to cold, fever and edema of the eyelids during the early stage, and systemic edema, joints pain, dysuria and floating pulse during the late stage. The treatment principle is to dispel wind, disperse Lung qi and promote urination.

❸ *Pi Shui**: Is a type of edema caused by excessive dampness with Spleen deficiency leading to effusion of fluids into the superficial layers. Manifestations are chronic onset, and include systemic and pitting edema, abdominal distention that is taut, no sweat nor thirst, and a floating pulse. The treatment principle is to strengthen the Spleen and transform dampness, facilitate the flow of yang qi and promote urination.

# Xi Xian Cao

*Herba Siegesbeckiae*
*Bitter, cold; Liver, Kidney*

[Characteristics] The raw herb is cold and effective in treating Damp-heat Painful Obstruction. After steamed with wine, this herb becomes sweet and warm and has the additional function of tonifying the Liver and Kidney.

| FUNCTIONS • INDICATIONS & MAJOR COMBINATIONS |
|---|
| **1. Dispel wind-dampness and unblock the channels:** <br> • Wind-dampness Painful Obstruction with heat. *+ Chou Wu Tong* <br> • Chronic wind-dampness accompanied by insufficiency of the Liver and Kidney. Steam this herb with wine for treating this condition. |
| **2. Clear heat and relieve toxicity:** <br> • Toxic swelling, sores, ulcers and eczema with itchy skin. *+ Bai Ji Li, Bai Xian Pi* |

[Dosage] 10-15 g. Raw herb is used for eczema, sores and ulcers; steam the herb with wine for painful obstruction.

# Sang Zhi

*Ramulus Mori*
*Bitter, neutral; Liver*

[Characteristics] Mainly entering the Liver channel, Sang Zhi dispels wind-dampness and unblocks the channels. It effectively treats painful obstruction affecting the upper extremities.

| FUNCTIONS • INDICATIONS & MAJOR COMBINATIONS |
|---|
| **1. Dispel wind-dampness and unblock the channels:** <br> • Wind-dampness Painful Obstruction, especially for those affecting the upper extremities. *+ Gui Zhi, Fang Feng* |
| **2. Promote urination and reduce swelling for edema.** |

[Dosage] 10-30 g.

[Comments] Both Sang Zhi and Gui Zhi facilitate the circulation in the collaterals. Sang Zhi dispels wind-dampness to unblock the channels; Gui Zhi warms yang qi to unblock the channels. Together they form the classic combination for Wind-dampness Painful Obstruction affecting the upper extremities.

# Luo Shi Teng

*Caulis Trachelospermi*
*Bitter, slightly cold; Heart, Liver*

[Characteristics] Bitter and slightly cold, Luo Shi Teng dispels wind-dampness and unblocks the channels; it is very useful in treating wind-damp-heat obstruction. It also cools the blood and reduces swelling.

| FUNCTIONS • INDICATIONS & MAJOR COMBINATIONS |
| --- |
| **1. Dispel wind-dampness and unblock the channels:** <br> • Wind-damp-heat Painful Obstruction with spasms of sinews. <br> *+ Ren Dong Teng, Sang Zhi* |
| **2. Cool the blood and reduce swelling:** <br> • Swollen sore throat. Sip the decoction of this single herb slowly. <br> • Toxic swelling, sores and carbuncles. *+ Gua Lou, Ru Xiang* |

[Dosage] 6-15 g.

# Hai Tong Pi

*Cortex Erythrinae*
*Bitter, acrid, neutral; Liver*

[Characteristics] Mainly entering the Liver channel, Hai Tong Pi has bitter, acrid and neutral properties. It tends to work well on the lower extremities, and it is useful in treating Wind-dampness Painful Obstruction attacking the lower back or knees. To stop itchiness, it is applied topically to dry dampness and dispel wind.

| FUNCTIONS • INDICATIONS & MAJOR COMBINATIONS |
| --- |
| **1. Dispel wind-dampness and unblock the channels:** <br> • Wind-dampness Painful Obstruction, especially for the lower extremities and lower back. *+ Niu Xi, Wu Jia Pi* |
| **2. Kill parasites to stop itchiness from eczema. Decoct the herb alone and use it as an external wash.** |

[Dosage] 6-15 g.

# Sang Ji Sheng

*Herba Taxilli*
*Bitter, neutral; Liver, Kidney*

[Characteristics] Bitter and neutral, moist in consistency, it dispels wind-dampness as well as tonifies the Liver and Kidney. Sang Ji Sheng is commonly used for painful obstruction and weakness of the sinews and bones due to either blood deficiency or insufficiency of the Liver and Kidney. In addition, it stabilizes the Penetrating and Conception vessels to calm the fetus.

| FUNCTIONS • INDICATIONS & MAJOR COMBINATIONS |
|---|
| **1. Dispel wind-dampness, augment the Liver and Kidney, and strengthen the sinews and bones:**<br>• Wind-dampness Painful Obstruction with soreness and weakness of the lower back and knees. *+ Du Huo, Du Zhong* |
| **2. Calm the fetus:**<br>• Insufficiency of the Liver and Kidney or instability of the Penetrating and Conception vessels with Restless Fetus Syndromes, and uterine bleeding during pregnancy. *+ E Jiao, Xu Duan* |

[Dosage] 10-30 g.

[Comments] Sang Ji Sheng predominately has a bitter property, which explains its primary function of expelling wind-dampness for the treatment of painful obstruction. Its secondary function is to tonify the Liver and Kidney. When treating insufficiency of the Liver and Kidney, it functions as an auxiliary herb, and is commonly combined with Du Zhong and Niu Xi, which have stronger functions to tonify the Liver and Kidney and strengthen the lower back and knees.

# Wu Jia Pi

*Cortex Acanthopanacis*
*Acrid, bitter, warm; Liver, Kidney*

**[Characteristics]** Dispels wind-dampness, as well as tonifies the Liver and Kidney to strengthen the sinews and bones. Wu Jia Pi is primarily used to treat Wind-dampness Painful Obstruction accompanied by weakness of the sinews and bones or delayed musculo-skeletal development in children. It also promotes urination and reduces swelling.

| FUNCTIONS • INDICATIONS & MAJOR COMBINATIONS |
| --- |

### 1. Dispel wind-dampness:
- Chronic Wind-dampness Painful Obstruction accompanied by insufficiency of the Liver and Kidney. Make a tincture of this herb alone, or *+ Mu Gua*

### 2. Strengthen the sinews and bones:
- Insufficiency of the Liver and Kidney with weakness of the sinews and bones. *+ Huai Niu Xi, Du Zhong*
- Delayed musculo-skeletal development in children. *+ Gui Ban, Niu Xi*

### 3. Promote urination and reduce swelling:
- *Pi Shui* due to excessive dampness with Spleen deficiency. *+ Fu Ling Pi, Da Fu Pi*

**[Dosage]** 6-10 g.

**[Comments]** ❶ Wu Jia Pi includes two types:

    **Nan Wu Jia**, non-toxic herb, is more powerful in dispelling wind-dampness, tonifying the Liver and Kidney, and strengthening the sinews and bones.

    **Bei Wu Jia**, toxic herb, has relatively stronger effects in promoting urination and reducing edema. Do not exceed the recommended dose.

    ❷ Traditionally, Wu Jia Pi is often prepared as a tincture to enhance its therapeutic effects.

# Qian Nian Jian

*Rhizoma Homalomenae*
*Acrid, bitter, warm; Liver, Kidney*

[Characteristics] Mainly enters the Liver and Kidney channels, Qian Nian Jian dispels wind-dampness and strengthens the sinews and bones. It is usually prepared as a tincture. This herb is especially useful for the elderly.

FUNCTIONS • INDICATIONS & MAJOR COMBINATIONS

**Dispel wind-dampness and strengthen the sinews and bones:**
- Wind-dampness Painful Obstruction with cold pain at the lower back and knees, and spasms or numbness at the lower extremities. Either use the tincture alone or *+ Gou Qi Zi, Niu Xi*

[Dosage] 6-10 g.

## [Remarks & Differentiations]

**Du Huo, Wei Ling Xian, Mu Gua, Hai Feng Teng and Bai Hua She:**
Warm in nature, they dispel wind-dampness and disperse cold, commonly used for Wind-dampness Painful Obstruction that is prone to cold.

**Qin Jiao, Fang Ji, Xi Xian Cao, Sang Zhi, Luo Shi Teng and Hai Tong Pi:**
Cold or cool in nature, they dispel wind-dampness and alleviate pain, especially effective for Wind-dampness Painful Obstruction with heat signs.

**Sang Ji Sheng, Wu Jia Pi and Qian Nian Jian:**
Dispel wind-dampness, as well as strengthen the sinews and bones, often used for chronic Wind-dampness Painful Obstruction accompanied by weakness of the sinews and bones.

# HERBS THAT
## Are Aromatic to Transform Dampness 5

Aromatic, they carry the effects of transforming dampness and reviving the Spleen, and treating turbid dampness lingering in the Spleen. Their characteristics are acrid, aromatic, warm and drying; they enter the Spleen and Stomach channels. The primary goal is to restore the function of transportation and transformation of the Spleen to treat dampness. The secondary goal is to make the qi flow smoothly in the middle burner. Herbs in this category are often used to treat dampness accumulated in the middle with epigastric and abdominal distention, fullness sensation and white greasy tongue coating. Damp-warm Febrile Disease can also be treated with these herbs.

Combine herbs that regulate the qi into the prescription to effectively treat dampness. Since there are two patterns of dampness, cold and heat types, the prescription is usually modified. For example, add herbs that warm the interior for patterns of cold-dampness and add herbs that clear heat and dry dampness for patterns of damp-heat. If dampness is complicated with Spleen and Stomach deficiency, herbs that tonify the qi and strengthen the Spleen should be added.

Injury to the yin and fluid may occur with warm and drying herbs from this section; use with caution in yin deficiency condition. It is important not to decoct these herbs for long because its aromatic effects will be diminished.

# Cang Zhu

*Rhizoma Atractylodis*
*Acrid, bitter, warm; Spleen, Stomach*

**[Characteristics]** Internally, it dries dampness to strengthen the Spleen and harmonize the Stomach. Cang Zhu is used as the primary herb for dampness accumulating in the middle burner with epigastric and abdominal distention, and thick greasy tongue coating. Externally, it releases the exterior and induces sweating to dispel wind-cold for exterior wind-cold condtions or Wind-cold-damp Painful Obstruction. It also enhances visual acuity.

**FUNCTIONS • INDICATIONS & MAJOR COMBINATIONS**

**1. Dry dampness and strengthen the Spleen:**
  • Dampness accumulating in the middle burner with distention in the epigastrium and abdomen, nausea and vomiting, poor appetite and thick greasy tongue coating. *+ Hou Po, Chen Pi*

**2. Dispel wind-dampness:**
  • Wind-cold-damp Painful Obstruction. *+ Du Huo, Qin Jiao*
  • Damp-heat infusing downward with weak, painful and swollen knees and feet. *+ Huang Bai*

**3. Release the exterior and disperse cold:**
  • Exterior wind-cold-dampness with aversion to cold, fever and general body ache. *+ Qiang Huo, Fang Feng*

**4. Improve visual acuity for night blindness.**

**[Dosage]** 6-10 g. Fried form is used to dry dampness and strengthen the Spleen; raw form is used to release the exterior and disperse cold.

**[Comments]** ❶A bitter and warm herb, Cang Zhu works well in drying dampness and is used to treat conditions related to cold-damp. However, when it is combined with Huang Bai, a bitter and cold herb, they can treat conditions associated with damp-heat infusing downward. It also can be used together with Shi Gao and Zhi Mu, extremely cold herbs, for Damp-warm Febrile Disease with fever, focal distention in the chest, sweating and thick greasy tongue coating. These combinations are used for clearing heat together with drying dampness.

❷ Cang Zhu and Bai Zhu are both from the Atractylodis family. They were used interchangeably in ancient time; however, today, they are considered to be unique and are used for different indications or purposes. For differentiation and application (p. 211).

# Hou Po

*Cortex Magnoliae Officinalis*
*Bitter, acrid, warm; Lung, Spleen, Stomach, Large Intestine*

[Characteristics] In addition to warming the middle and drying dampness, Hou Po possesses the function of facilitating the flow of qi. It can disperse the insubstantial formation of cold-dampness and qi stagnations, as well as relieve the substantial accumulation of food and phlegm. It is primarily used for disharmony of the Spleen and Stomach with focal distention in the epigastrium and abdomen due to dampness accumulation, food retention and qi stagnation.

---

**FUNCTIONS • INDICATIONS & MAJOR COMBINATIONS**

**1. Dry dampness and relieve focal distention:**
- Dampness accumulating in the middle burner. *+ Cang Zhu, Chen Pi*
- Middle burner deficient cold with distention. *+ Ren Shen, Gan Cao*
- Cold-dampness injuring the Spleen and Stomach with abdominal distention and pain. *+ Gan Jiang, Cao Dou Kou*

**2. Promote the movement of qi and reduce the accumulations:**
- Food retention and qi stagnation or heat accumulation with fecal impaction, abdominal distention and pain. *+ Da Huang, Zhi Shi*

**3. Transform phlegm and calm wheezing:**
- Exterior-contracted wind-cold with pre-existing wheezing. *+ Xing Ren, Gui Zhi*
- Pattern of excess above and deficiency below with coughing, wheezing and shortness of breath. *+ Ban Xia, Qian Hu*
- Plum-pit Syndromes. *+ Ban Xia, Zi Su Ye*

---

[Dosage] 3-10 g.

[Comments] To emphasize its bitter and warm nature and dry dampness effect, Hou Po is categorized into the herbs that are aromatic to transform dampness. Recognizing its strong dispersing and moving effects, it is known as the primary herb for reducing distention and eliminating fullness. Therefore, it is a common herb for treating focal distention in the epigastrium and abdomen due to cold types of pathogenic factors obstructing the flow of qi. For damp obstruction and qi stagnation, Hou Po is often combined with Cang Zhu. To treat phlegm with constrained qi, Ban Xia is added. To treat fecal impaction due to heat accumulation, Hou Po is used with Zhi Shi. Based on its strength of facilitating the flow of qi, Hou Po is also classified into the herbs that regulate the qi in some traditional textbooks.

**Herbs that are Aromatic to Transform Dampness**

# Huo Xiang

*Herba Pogostemonis*
*Acrid, slightly warm; Spleen, Stomach, Lung*

[Characteristics] An aromatic herb with the effect of transforming dampness, it can harmonize the middle burner and stop vomiting; it is also an acrid herb with the effect of dispersing to release the exterior and relieve summerheat. Huo Xiang is the primary herb for the treatment of summerheat-dampness with aversion to cold, fever, focal distention in the chest and diaphragm, vomiting and diarrhea.

| FUNCTIONS • INDICATIONS & MAJOR COMBINATIONS |
| --- |
| **1. Transform dampness:**<br>• Dampness accumulating in the middle burner. *+ Cang Zhu, Hou Po* |
| **2. Relieve summerheat and release the exterior:**<br>• Exterior wind-cold in summer and internal injuries by cold or raw food with aversion to cold, fever, vomiting and diarrhea. *+ Zi Su Ye*<br>• Early stage of Damp-warm Febrile Disease. *+ Hua Shi, Huang Qin* |
| **3. Stop vomiting:**<br>• For all patterns of vomiting.<br>— Dampness hindering the middle burner. *+ Ban Xia*<br>— Damp-heat hindering the middle burner. *+ Huang Lian*<br>— Spleen and Stomach deficiency. *+ Dang Shen, Gan Cao*<br>— Morning sickness. *+ Sha Ren, Ban Xia* |

[Dosage] 6-10 g. May double the dose when using the fresh herb.

[Comments] ❶ Different parts of this plant have their unique features and therapeutic effects such as:

**Huo Xiang Ye**, the leaf of Huo Xiang, is more effective in dispersing and releasing the exterior.

**Huo Xiang Geng**, the stem of Huo Xiang, is more effective in harmonizing the middle burner and stopping vomiting.

**Xian Huo Xiang**, the fresh herb that is mildly drying, is more effective in relieving summerheat and transforming dampness.

❷ Both Huo Xiang and Zi Su can dispel the pathogenic factors and release the exterior, facilitate the flow of qi and harmonize the middle. However, the former has stronger aromatic and drying properties to effectively transform dampness and stop vomiting; while the latter has stronger acrid and dispersing qualities to induce perspiration and disperse cold.

# Pei Lan

*Herba Eupatorii*
*Acrid, neutral; Spleen, Stomach*

**[Characteristics]** Pei Lan eliminates the excessive turbid dampness that lingers in the middle burner with good effect. It is therefore an important herb for sweet taste or sticky sensation in the mouth due to dampness hindering the middle burner. It is also used to treat exterior conditions of summerheat-dampness.

| FUNCTIONS • INDICATIONS & MAJOR COMBINATIONS |
| --- |
| **1. Transform dampness:** <br> • Dampness accumulating in the middle burner with sweet taste or sticky sensation in the mouth. *+ Huo Xiang, Cang Zhu* |
| **2. Relieve summerheat:** <br> • Exterior conditions of summerheat-dampness. *+ Huo Xiang, He Ye* <br> • Early stage of Damp-warm Febrile Disease. *+ Hua Shi, Yi Yi Ren* |

**[Dosage]** 6-10 g. Double the dose when using the fresh herb.


# Sha Ren

*Fructus Amomi*
*Acrid, warm; Spleen, Stomach*

**[Characteristics]** An important herb to transform dampness, facilitate the qi flow and harmonize the Spleen and Stomach, it is used for dampness accumulating in the middle with qi stagnation. It also facilitates the flow of qi to calm the fetus.

| FUNCTIONS • INDICATIONS & MAJOR COMBINATIONS |
| --- |
| **1. Transform dampness and facilitate the flow of qi:** <br> • Dampness accumulating in the middle burner with Spleen and Stomach qi stagnation. *+ Hou Po, Cang Zhu* <br> • Spleen deficiency with qi stagnation. *+ Dang Shen, Bai Zhu* |
| **2. Calm the fetus:** <br> • Spleen deficiency accompanied by qi stagnation with Restless Fetus Syndromes. *+ Bai Zhu, Zi Su Geng* |
| **3. Warm the middle burner for cold-dampness with diarrhea.** |

**[Dosage]** 3-6 g. Add Sha Ren to the decoction towards the end.

**Herbs that are Aromatic to Transform Dampness**

# Bai Dou Kou

*Fructus Amomi Rotundus*
*Acrid, warm; Spleen, Stomach, Lung*

[Characteristics] It is aromatic to transform dampness from the middle burner as well as promote the flow of qi in the Spleen and Stomach. Bai Dou Kou is used for Spleen and Stomach qi stagnation due to dampness accumulation, vomiting due to cold in the Stomach, and early stage of Damp-warm Febrile Disease.

**FUNCTIONS • INDICATIONS & MAJOR COMBINATIONS**

### 1. Transform dampness and facilitate the flow of qi:
  - Dampness hindering the Spleen and Stomach. *+ Cang Zhu, Hou Po*
  - Early stage of Damp-warm Febrile Disease with stifling sensation in the chest, loss of appetite and greasy tongue coating.
    — Excessive dampness. *+ Xing Ren, Yi Yi Ren*
    — Excessive heat. *+ Huang Qin, Huang Lian*

### 2. Warm the middle and stop vomiting:
  - Cold-dampness accumulating in the Stomach with vomiting.
    *+ Huo Xiang, Ban Xia*

[Dosage] 3-6 g. Add to the decoction towards the end.


# Cao Dou Kou

*Semen Alpiniae Katsumadai*
*Acrid, warm; Spleen, Stomach*

[Characteristics] In comparison to Bai Dou Kou, Cao Dou Kou shares the same functions of drying dampness and facilitating the flow of qi; however, in terms of their strengthes, Cao Dou Kou has a stronger function of drying damp and a weaker function in regulating qi flow. It also warms the middle burner.

**FUNCTIONS • INDICATIONS & MAJOR COMBINATIONS**

### Dry dampness, facilitate the flow of qi and warm the middle burner:
  - Cold-dampness hindering the Spleen and Stomach with distention and pain in the epigastrium and abdomen, vomiting and diarrhea.
    — Excessive dampness. *+ Hou Po, Cang Zhu*
    — Excessive cold. *+ Rou Gui, Gan Jiang*

[Dosage] 3-6 g. It is recommended to add this herb to the decoction near the end.

# Cao Guo

*Fructus Tsaoko*
*Acrid, warm; Spleen, Stomach*

[Characteristics] Extremely warm and drying, Cao Guo is used for severe cases of cold-dampness accumulating in the middle burner. It also keeps malarial disorder under control.

| FUNCTIONS • INDICATIONS & MAJOR COMBINATIONS |
| --- |

**1. Dry dampness and warm the middle burner:**
- Cold-dampness accumulating in the middle burner. *+ Hou Po, Cang Zhu*

**2. Keep malarial disorder under control:**
- Malaria in which there is excessive cold-dampness. *+ Chang Shan, Chai Hu*

[Dosage] 3-6 g.

## [Remarks & Differentiations]

### Sha Ren, Bai Dou Kou, Cao Dou Kou and Cao Guo:

They all share the basic functions of transforming dampness and facilitating the flow of qi.

As listed in the order from left to right, the strength of transforming dampness increases, while the effects of facilitating the flow of qi decreases. Therefore, among these four herbs, Cao Guo has the strongest strength in transforming dampness, and Sha Ren has the best effect in facilitating the movement of qi.

**Herbs that are Aromatic to Transform Dampness**

# HERBS THAT
## Drain Dampness 6

The functions of these herbs are to unblock the obstruction and regulate the flow of water passage to drain dampness. Most herbs in this category are sweet and bland to leach out dampness or bitter and cold to descend and drain dampness. They enter the Bladder, Spleen and Kidney channels to diurese, regulate the smooth flow of urine, and drain the accumulated dampness by way of urination. Some herbs also clear heat and drain dampness or eliminate jaundice. They are usually used for the treatment of dysuria, edema, congested fluids, Painful Urinary Dysfunction, jaundice and Damp-warm Febrile Disease.

When preparing the formula, remember to treat the origin of dampness. For example, combine herbs that augment the qi and warm the yang when treating edema due to yang deficiency; add herbs that clear heat, unblock the obstruction in the urinary tract, or cool the blood and stop bleeding to treat Heat-type or Blood-type of Painful Urinary Dysfunction, and add herbs that disperse Lung qi and induce sweating in early stage of edema with exterior condition.

Use these herbs with caution in yin deficiency or body fluid insufficiency. Inappropriate use of these herbs may lead to depletion of the fluid.

# Fu Ling

*Poria*
*Sweet, bland, neutral; Heart, Spleen, Kidney*

[Characteristics] Sweet, bland and neutral, Fu Ling tonifies the middle burner and leaches out dampness. With the combination of sweet and bland, it is neither an aggressive tonic nor a harsh drainer, but rather a gentle herb; it evenly tonifies the righteous qi as well as expels the pathogenic factors. Fu Ling is the imperial herb for Spleen deficiency with excessive dampness causing congested fluids, edema and diarrhea. It also strengthens the Spleen, quiets the Heart and calms the spirit.

| FUNCTIONS • INDICATIONS & MAJOR COMBINATIONS |
|---|
| **1. Promote urination and leach out dampness:** |
| • Patterns of dampness with dysuria and edema. *+ Zhu Ling, Ze Xie* |
|   — Damp-heat. *+ Che Qian Zi, Mu Tong* |
|   — Cold-damp. *+ Fu Zi, Gan Jiang* |
| • Accumulation of congested fluids with palpitation, dizziness and cough. *+ Bai Zhu, Gui Zhi* |
| **2. Strengthen the Spleen:** |
| • Spleen deficiency with fatigue and poor appetite. *+ Dang Shen* |
| **3. Quiet the restless Heart and calm the spirit:** |
| • Palpitation, restlessness and insomnia. *+ Suan Zao Ren, Yuan Zhi* |

[Dosage] 10-15 g. Stir with Zhu Sha for the function of calming the spirit.

[Comments] Different parts of the plant have their unique features and therapeutic effects such as:

      **Bai Fu Ling**, the white central portion of the sclerotium, has the therapeutic effect of strengthening the Spleen.

      **Chi Fu Ling**, the slightly red portion underneath the peel of the sclerotium, tends to drain dampness.

      **Fu Shen**, the white part that grows around the root, known as Bao Mu Fu Shen, is more effective in calming the spirit.

## [Addendum]
## Fu Ling Pi
### *Cortex Poria*
Has the same properties as Fu Ling, Fu Ling Pi promotes urination and reduces swelling. It is primarily used to treat edema, and commonly combined with Sheng Jiang Pi and Da Fu Pi. 10-15 g.

# Zhu Ling

*Polyporus*
*Sweet, bland, neutral; Kidney, Bladder*

[**Characteristics**] Sweet, bland and neutral, it enters the lower burner, Kidney and Bladder. Zhu Ling exclusively promotes urination and reduces edema without having any tonifying effect.

**FUNCTIONS • INDICATIONS & MAJOR COMBINATIONS**

**Promote urination and leach out dampness:**
- Spleen deficiency with edema and dysuria. *+ Fu Ling, Ze Xie*
- Yin deficiency with heat accompanied by water-heat complex with dysuria and edema. *+ E Jiao, Hua Shi*

[**Dosage**] 6-10 g.


# Ze Xie

*Rhizoma Alismatis*
*Sweet, bland, cold; Kidney, Bladder*

[**Characteristics**] Sweet, bland and cold in nature, bland to leach out dampness, Ze Xie enters the Bladder to promote urination and reduce swelling; cold to drain heat, it enters the Kidney to drain *Xiang Huo* and eliminate deficient heat. It is commonly used for damp-heat accumulation with dysuria, edema and diarrhea, as well as yin deficiency with five palms heat and night sweating.

**FUNCTIONS • INDICATIONS & MAJOR COMBINATIONS**

**1. Promote urination and leach out dampness:**
- Dysfunction of the Bladder to transform qi with edema and dysuria. *+ Fu Ling, Zhu Ling*
- Spleen deficiency with excessive dampness or congested fluids with dizziness. *+ Bai Zhu*

**2. Drain heat:**
- Damp-heat infusing downward with Painful Urinary Dysfunction or excessive vaginal discharge. *+ Huang Bai, Che Qian Zi*
- Kidney yin insufficiency with five palms heat, night sweating and tinnitus. *+ Shu Di Huang, Mu Dan Pi*

[**Dosage**] 6-10 g.

**Herbs that Drain Dampness**

*long-term can cause miscarriage —*
*avoid during pregnancy*

# Yi Yi Ren

*Semen Coicis*
*Sweet, bland, slightly cold; Spleen, Stomach, Lung*

[Characteristics] Bland in nature, this herb leaches out dampness; sweet in nature, it augments the Spleen. Yi Yi Ren has a gentle action and its primary functions are strengthening the Spleen and draining dampness. It can be used for all patterns of edema and diarrhea due to Spleen deficiency with excessive dampness. Yi Yi Ren is also effective in eliminating dampness from the sinews and muscles; therefore, it is commonly used to treat painful obstruction with spasms of the sinews with good results. Additionally, it is often used for Lung abscess and intestinal abscess.

**FUNCTIONS • INDICATIONS & MAJOR COMBINATIONS**

### 1. Strengthen the Spleen, promote urination and leach out dampness:
- Spleen deficiency causing excessive dampness with edema and dysuria. *+ Fu Ling, Zhu Ling*
- Spleen deficiency with diarrhea, poor appetite and abdominal distention. *+ Dang Shen, Bai Zhu*
- Qi level of Damp-warm Febrile Disease with excessive dampness. *+ Xing Ren, Bai Dou Kou*

### 2. Drain damp-heat:
- Damp-heat infusing downward with red swollen painful knees and feet which are warm to touch or excessive vaginal discharge and external genital itchiness. *+ Cang Zhu, Huang Bai*

### 3. Relieve painful obstruction:
- Wind-dampness Painful Obstruction with spasms of the sinews. *+ Ma Huang, Xing Ren*

### 4. Clear heat and promote purulent discharge:
- Lung abscess. *+ Tao Ren, Lu Gen*
- Intestinal abscess. *+ Bai Jiang Cao, Mu Dan Pi*

[Dosage] 10-30 g. Frying this herb to increase the effect of strengthening the Spleen, raw for other purposes.

[Comments] With its gentle action, Yi Yi Ren should be used in large doses and for long periods of time. As a therapeutic nutritional supplement, it is often cooked into porridge with Jing Mi.

# Che Qian Zi

*Semen Plantaginis*
*Sweet, cold; Kidney, Liver, Lung*

[Characteristics] This herb specifically descends, drains and directs the fluid to flow smoothly. Che Qian Zi descends and eliminates damp-heat via urination. Therefore, it is commonly used for damp-heat with edema, Painful Urinary Dysfunction and diarrhea. It also clears and drains heat from the Lung and Liver to treat Lung heat with cough and Liver heat with red eyes.

| FUNCTIONS • INDICATIONS & MAJOR COMBINATIONS |
|---|
| **1. Clear heat, promote urination and unblock the obstruction of the urinary tract:**<br>• Edema and dysuria. *+ Fu Ling, Zhu Ling*<br>• Painful Urinary Dysfunction due to damp-heat in the Bladder. *+ Mu Tong, Zhi Zi* |
| **2. Stop diarrhea:**<br>• Excessive dampness with diarrhea. May use the powdered form alone, or *+ Bai Zhu, Fu Ling* |
| **3. Clear heat from the Liver and enhance visual acuity:**<br>• Liver heat with red swollen painful eyes. *+ Ju Hua, Huang Qin*<br>• Liver and Kidney yin deficiency with blurry vision. *+ Gou Qi Zi, Di Huang* |
| **4. For Lung heat cough, it is usually combined with herbs that clear heat and transform phlegm.** |

[Dosage] 6-10 g. Seal in tea bags for decoction.

[Comments] Che Qian Zi has a unique characteristic of unblocking the water passage and separating the clear from the turbid. It is commonly used to treat watery diarrhea due to excessive dampness, namely, "promoting urination to solidify the bowel movements".

# Hua Shi

*Talcum*
*Sweet, bland, cold; Stomach, Bladder*

[Characteristics] Mainly clears and eliminates damp-heat from the Bladder to promote urination and unblock the obstruction of the urinary tract. It also relieves summerheat to treat irritability and intense thirst during the summer.

| FUNCTIONS • INDICATIONS & MAJOR COMBINATIONS |
| --- |
| **1. Clear heat and unblock the obstruction of the urinary tract:**<br>• Painful Urinary Dysfunction due to damp-heat in the Bladder.<br>  *+ Mu Tong, Che Qian Zi* |
| **2. Relieve summerheat:**<br>• Summerheat with irritability and intense thirst. *+ Gan Cao* |
| **3. For skin disorders related to dampness, such as eczema, apply topically.** |

[Dosage] 10-15 g. Seal in tea bags for decoction.

# Mu Tong

*Caulis Aristolochiae Manshuriensis*
*Bitter, cold; Heart, Small Intestine, Bladder*

[Characteristics] Mu Tong acts on the upper organs together with the lower organs to clear heat from the Heart while drain dampness from the Small Intestine and Bladder. It is used for irritability with scanty dark urine, and Painful Urinary Dysfunction due to damp-heat in the Bladder. It also promotes lactation.

| FUNCTIONS • INDICATIONS & MAJOR COMBINATIONS |
| --- |
| **1. Clear heat and unblock the obstruction of the urinary tract:**<br>• Damp-heat type of Painful Urinary Dysfunction. *+ Zhi Zi, Hua Shi*<br>• Heart fire shifted to the Small Intestine with irritability, sores in the mouth and tongue, and scanty dark urine. *+ Zhu Ye, Sheng Di Huang* |
| **2. Promote lactation for post-partum insufficient lactation.** |
| **3. Damp-heat Painful Obstruction.** |

[Dosage] 3-6 g.

[Precautions] Acute renal failure may result from overdose. It is not recommended to use in large doses nor for long-term usage. Contraindicated during pregnancy.

# Tong Cao

*Medulla Tetrapanacis*
*Sweet, bland, slightly cold; Lung, Stomach*

**[Characteristics]** Having both ascending and descending actions, Tong Cao guides the heat downward to unblock the obstruction of the urinary tract, as well as enters the Stomach to lift the flow of qi to promote lactation.

### FUNCTIONS • INDICATIONS & MAJOR COMBINATIONS

**1. Clear heat and unblock the obstruction of the urinary tract:**
  • Painful Urinary Dysfunction due to damp-heat. *+ Che Qian Zi*

**2. Promote lactation:**
  • Post-partum insufficient lactation. *+ Wang Bu Liu Xing*

**[Dosage]** 3-6 g.

**[Precautions]** Use with caution during pregnancy.

**[Comments]** For clarifications, the Tong Cao in ancient literature is the Mu Tong used in modern application; and the Tong Tuo Mu in ancient literature is the Tong Cao used in modern application.


# Deng Xin Cao

*Medulla Junci*
*Sweet, bland, slightly cold; Heart, Lung, Small Intestine*

**[Characteristics]** With similar yet milder effects of promoting urination and unblocking the obstruction of the urinary tract as Mu Tong, Deng Xin Cao also enters the Heart channel to clear heat from the Heart and eliminate irritability.

### FUNCTIONS • INDICATIONS & MAJOR COMBINATIONS

**1. Clear heat and unblock the obstruction of the urinary tract:**
  • Mild cases of Heat-type of Painful Urinary Dysfunction.

**2. Clear heat from the Heart and eliminate irritability:**
  • Heat in the Heart channel in childhood with night terrors and crying.

**3. External spray to treat obstructive pharyngolaryngeal inflammation.**

**[Dosage]** 1-3 g. To clear the Heart and eliminate irritability, stir in this herb with Zhu Sha; calcine and powder this herb for external application.

# Bi Xie

*Rhizoma Dioscoreae Septemlobae*
*Bitter, neutral; Liver, Stomach, Bladder*

**[Characteristics]** Bi Xie is effective in draining dampness to separate the clear from the turbid. It is used for damp turbidities infusing downward with cloudy urination, excessive vaginal discharge, as well as for Wind-damp Painful Obstruction.

**FUNCTIONS • INDICATIONS & MAJOR COMBINATIONS**

**1. Promote urination and separate the clear from the turbid:**
- Painful Urinary Dysfunction with cloudy urination. *+ Shi Chang Pu, Wu Yao*
- Damp turbidities infusing downward with excessive vaginal discharge. *+ Cang Zhu, Qian Shi*

**2. Expel wind-dampness:**
- Wind-dampness Painful Obstruction.

**[Dosage]** 10-15 g.

# Shi Wei

*Folium Pyrrosiae*
*Bitter, sweet, slightly cold; Bladder, Lung*

**[Characteristics]** Promoting urination and unblocking the obstruction of the urinary tract, Shi Wei can cool the blood and stop bleeding; therefore, it is often used for Painful Urinary Dysfunction of Heat or Blood type. It also clears heat from the Lung and stops coughing.

**FUNCTIONS • INDICATIONS & MAJOR COMBINATIONS**

**1. Promote urination and unblock the obstruction of the urinary tract:**
- Painful Urinary Dysfunction of Heat, Blood or Stone type. *+ Zhi Zi, Pu Huang*

**2. Clear heat from the Lung and stop coughing:**
- Lung heat with coughing, wheezing or asthma.

**3. Use for heat causing reckless movement of the blood with hematemesis, subcutaneous and mucosa bleeding.**

**[Dosage]** 6-10 g.

# Bian Xu

*Herba Polygoni Avicularis*
*Bitter, slightly cold; Bladder*

[Characteristics] Promoting urination and unblocking the obstruction of the urinary tract, Bian Xu is used for Damp-heat-type of Painful Urinary Dysfunction. It also kills parasites and stops itchiness with topical applications.

| FUNCTIONS • INDICATIONS & MAJOR COMBINATIONS |
|---|
| **1. Promote urination and unblock the obstruction of the urinary tract:** |
| • Damp-heat-type of Painful Urinary Dysfunction. *+ Qu Mai, Hua Shi* |
| • Blood-type of Painful Urinary Dysfunction. *+ Da Ji, Bai Mao Gen* |
| **2. Kill the parasites and stop itchiness:** |
| • Skin disorders due to dampness with eczema or genital itchiness. External wash with the decoction. |

[Dosage] 10-15 g.


# Qu Mai

*Herba Dianthi*
*Bitter, cold; Bladder, Heart, Small Intestine*

[Characteristics] Promoting urination and unblocking the obstruction of the urinary tract, Qu Mai is used for Painful Urinary Dysfunction. It also invigorates the blood and facilitates the menstrual flow for amenorrhea due to blood stasis.

| FUNCTIONS • INDICATIONS & MAJOR COMBINATIONS |
|---|
| **1. Promote urination and unblock the obstruction of the urinary tract:** |
| • Damp-heat-type of Painful Urinary Dysfunction. *+ Bian Xu, Hua Shi* |
| **2. Invigorate the blood and facilitate the menstrual flow:** |
| • Blood stasis with amenorrhea. *+ Tao Ren, Hong Hua* |

[Dosage] 10-15 g.

[Precautions] Contraindicated during pregnancy.

# Di Fu Zi

*Fructus Kochiae*
*Bitter, cold; Bladder*

[Characteristics] Promoting urination and clearing heat with mild effects, Di Fu Zi works more effectively in eliminating damp-heat and stopping itchiness for skin disorders due to dampness.

**FUNCTIONS • INDICATIONS & MAJOR COMBINATIONS**

**1. Clear heat and promote urination:**
  • Used as an auxiliary herb for Painful Urinary Dysfunction.

**2. Eliminate dampness and stop itchiness:**
  • Skin disorders due to dampness with itchiness.
    — Oral administration. *+ Huang Bai, Bai Xian Pi*
    — External wash. *+ Ku Shen, She Chuang Zi*

[Dosage] 10-15 g.

# Chi Xiao Dou

*Semen Phaseoli*
*Sweet, sour, neutral; Heart, Small Intestine*

[Characteristics] Promotes urination and reduces swelling for conditions of edema, as well as clears heat and relieves toxicity for heat toxicity with sores and abscesses. It also drains dampness and eliminates jaundice.

**FUNCTIONS • INDICATIONS & MAJOR COMBINATIONS**

**1. Promote urination and reduce swelling:**
  • Edema. May be used alone, or *+ Bai Mao Gen, Sang Bai Pi*

**2. Relieve toxicity and promote purulent discharge:**
  • Breast abscess, mumps and erysipelas. May be applied topically.

**3. Drain dampness and eliminate jaundice for damp-heat jaundice.**

[Dosage] 10-30 g.

# Yin Chen Hao

*Herba Artemisiae Scopariae*
*Bitter, slightly cold; Liver, Gallbladder, Spleen, Stomach*

[Characteristics] Exclusively drains dampness, clears heat and eliminates jaundice; Yin Chen Hao is the imperial herb for jaundice. With appropriate combinations, it is used to treat all patterns of jaundice regardless of yang or yin types.

| FUNCTIONS • INDICATIONS & MAJOR COMBINATIONS |
|---|
| **1. Drain dampness, clear heat and eliminate jaundice:** <br> • Yang-type jaundice. <br> — Heat predominates. *+ Da Huang, Zhi Zi* <br> — Dampness predominates. *+ Zhu Ling, Fu Ling* <br> • Yin-type jaundice. *+ Fu Zi, Gan Jiang* |
| **2. For skin disorders due to dampness with itchiness and oozing of yellow exudate, take the oral form or use the external wash.** |

[Dosage] 10-30 g.


# Jin Qian Cao

*Herba Lysimachiae*
*Sweet, bland, neutral; Liver, Gallbladder, Kidney, Bladder*

[Characteristics] Drains dampness, clears heat and eliminates jaundice; Jin Qian Cao softens hardness and expels calculi. It is the imperial herb for urinary and biliary calculi.

| FUNCTIONS • INDICATIONS & MAJOR COMBINATIONS |
|---|
| **1. Promote urination and unblock the obstruction of the urinary tract:** <br> • Painful Urinary Dysfunction of Heat or Stone type. *+ Ji Nei Jin, Hai Jin Sha* |
| **2. Drain dampness and eliminate jaundice:** <br> • Damp-heat jaundice. *+ Yin Chen Hao, Zhi Zi* <br> • Biliary calculi. *+ Yu Jin, Chai Hu* |
| **3. To relieve toxicity and to reduce the swelling from toxic sores, apply the fresh herb topically.** |

[Dosage] 30-60 g. May double the dose when using the fresh herb.

**Herbs that Drain Dampness**

## [Remarks & Differentiations]

**Fu Ling, Zhu Ling, Ze Xie and Yi Yi Ren:**

These herbs are sweet, bland and neutral or slightly cold. With bland property, they effectively leach out dampness to promote urination and reduce edema.

**Che Qian Zi, Hua Shi, Mu Tong, Tong Cao, Deng Xin Cao, Bi Xie, Shi Wei, Bian Xu, Qu Mai, and Di Fu Zi:**

All are cold herbs; they can promote urination as well as clear heat for Damp-heat-type of Painful Urinary Dysfunction.

**Yin Chen Hao and Jin Qian Cao:**

Both can clear heat, drain dampness, and eliminate jaundice for damp-heat jaundice.

### Fu Ling — Zhu Ling

|   | **Fu Ling** | **Zhu Ling** |
|---|---|---|
| **C** | Promote urination and leach out dampness for edema and dysuria. | |
| **D** | • Strengthens the Spleen and augments the qi for Spleen deficiency with excessive dampness. <br>• Quiets the restless Heart and calms the spirit. | • Exclusively promotes urination without having any tonifying effect. |

### Fu Ling — Yi Yi Ren

|   | **Fu Ling** | **Yi Yi Ren** |
|---|---|---|
| **C** | Strengthen the Spleen, promote urination and leach out dampness. | |
| **D** | • Sweet and neutral, enters the Heart to quiet the restless Heart and calm the spirit. | • Slightly cold, clears heat and promotes purulent discharge for Lung abscess, etc. <br>• Eliminates dampness from the sinews and muscles for painful obstruction. |

**Herbs that Drain Dampness**

## Mu Tong — Deng Xin Cao

| | Mu Tong | Deng Xin Cao |
|---|---|---|
| C | Clear heat and unblock the obstruction of the urinary tract. Enter the Heart channel to clear and drain heat. | |
| D | • Bitter and cold to strongly clear and drain Heart fire for Heart fire blazing up with sores in the mouth and tongue.<br>• Promotes lactation.<br><br>• Drains damp-heat to treat painful obstruction. | • Sweet, bland and slightly cold to mildly clear and drain Heart fire for childhood night terrors and crying.<br>• External spray for obstructive pharyngolaryngeal inflammation. |

## Shi Wei — Bian Xu — Qu Mai

| | Shi Wei | Bian Xu | Qu Mai |
|---|---|---|---|
| C | Promote urination and unblock the obstruction of the urinary tract. Combined for effect of mutual reinforcement. Painful Urinary Dysfunction of Heat or Blood type. | | |
| D | • Clears heat from the Lung and stops coughing. | • External application for eradicating parasites and stopping itchiness. | • Invigorates the blood and facilitates the menstrual flow. |

# HERBS THAT
## Transform Phlegm and Stop Coughing     7

To resolve phlegm, stop coughing and calm wheezing are the primary functions of herbs from this category. These herbs are further subcategorized into the following three groups: (1) herbs that warm and transform cold-phlegm, (2) herbs that clear and transform phlegm-heat, and (3) herbs that stop coughing and calm wheezing. They are used to treat various phlegm patterns including cold-phlegm, phlegm-dampness, phlegm-heat and wind-phlegm. Coughing and wheezing due to exterior or interior causes or goiter, scrofula and yin-type gangrene due to phlegm can also be treated with herbs in this category.

Coughing and wheezing are often accompanied with phlegm. Conversely, excessive phlegm induces coughing and wheezing in most instances. These herbs usually have the dual functions to transform phlegm as well as stop coughing and wheezing. In clinical practice, it is common to combine the group of herbs that transform phlegm with the group of herbs that stop coughing and calm wheezing.

Herbs that are warm and drying are contraindicated for use in yin deficiency with dry cough and hemoptysis; herbs that are cool and moist are contraindicated for use in patterns of cold-phlegm or phlegm-dampness.

# Ban Xia

*Rhizoma Pinelliae*
*Acrid, warm, toxic; Lung, Spleen, Stomach*

**[Characteristics]** It dries dampness, transforms phlegm, harmonizes the Stomach and descends the rebellious qi. Warm and drying in nature, Ban Xia is the imperial herb for treating phlegm-dampness due to Spleen failing to transform and transport water, and for dampness obstruction causing qi to rebel.

**FUNCTIONS • INDICATIONS & MAJOR COMBINATIONS**

**1. Dry dampness and transform phlegm:**
- Impaired transporting and transforming function of Spleen qi causing excessive dampness with copious sputum. *+ Chen Pi, Fu Ling*
  — Cold-type with thin white sputum. *+ Xi Xin, Gan Jiang*
  — Heat-type with viscous yellow sputum. *+ Huang Qin, Bei Mu*

**2. Harmonize the Stomach, descend rebellious qi and stop vomiting:**
- Rebellious Stomach qi with nausea and vomiting.
  — Cold congested fluids in the Stomach. *+ Sheng Jiang*
  — Heat in the Stomach. *+ Huang Lian*
  — Morning sickness. *+ Zi Su Geng*

**3. Reduce focal distention and dissipate nodules:**
- Heat-cold complex with chest and epigastric focal distention, and absence of pain upon palpation. *+ Gan Jiang, Huang Lian*
- Phlegm-heat with focal distention in the chest and epigastrium, and pain upon palpation. *+ Huang Lian, Gua Lou*
- Plum-pit Syndromes. *+ Hou Po, Zi Su Ye*
- For toxic swelling, sores and abscesses, apply the raw form topically.

**[Dosage]** 6-10 g. Mix the powdered form with wine for topical application.

**[Precautions]** Incompatible with Wu Tou. Use with caution in yin deficiency.

**[Comments]** ❶ The good quality herbs are the ones that have been stored for a long time; therefore, the alternative name is Chen Ban Xia, or aged Ban Xia.

❷ Raw Ban Xia is toxic; for clinical usage, Ban Xia is processed in various forms. The common forms are:

**Qing Ban Xia** is effective in transforming phlegm.

**Jiang Ban Xia** tends to have a better effect in stopping vomiting.

**Fa Ban Xia** dries dampness and strengthens the Spleen.

**Ban Xia Qu** transforms phlegm and relieves food stagnation.

# Tian Nan Xing

*Rhizoma Arisaematis*
*Bitter, acrid, warm, toxic; Liver, Lung, Spleen*

[Characteristics] Has similar effects as Ban Xia in drying dampness and transforming phlegm. However, it is extremely bitter, acrid, warm and much more drying. Tian Nan Xing mainly enters the Liver channel and specifically acts on the meridians; it is the primary herb used to treat wind-phlegm with dizziness, vertigo, facial paralysis and numbness of the extremities.

| FUNCTIONS • INDICATIONS & MAJOR COMBINATIONS |
| --- |

**1. Dry dampness and transform phlegm:**
- Stubborn cough and stifling sensation in the chest.
  — Phlegm-dampness. *+ Chen Pi, Ban Xia*
  — Phlegm-heat. *+ Huang Qin, Gua Lou*

**2. Expel wind-phlegm and alleviate tremors:**
- Wind-phlegm with dizziness. *+ Tian Ma, Ban Xia*
- Wind-phlegm obstructing the meridians with numbness of the limbs and hemiplegia. *+ Ban Xia, Bai Fu Zi*
- Tetanus. *+ Fang Feng, Bai Zhi*

**3. For sores, abscesses and toxic swelling, the raw form is often applied topically. It has an anti-neoplastic effect and may be used as an herbal supplement to treat cervical carcinoma.**

[Dosage] 6-10 g. Process before oral administration; raw herb is for topical application only.

[Precautions] Contraindicated during pregnancy, and for those of yin deficiency with dry cough.

[Addendum]
## Dan Nan Xing
*Arisaema cum Bile*
Bitter and cool, it clears heat, transforms phlegm, extinguishes wind and alleviates convulsions; it is primarily used for phlegm-heat with cough, and phlegm-heat with contractions, seizures, convulsions and manic behaviors.

# Bai Fu Zi

*Rhizoma Typhonii*
*Acrid, sweet, warm, toxic; Liver, Spleen, Stomach*

[Characteristics] When it disperses and ascends, it has a strong effect to expel wind-phlegm from the head for facial paralysis status post stroke and for treating headaches. It can also relieve toxicity and dissipate nodules.

**FUNCTIONS • INDICATIONS & MAJOR COMBINATIONS**

### 1. Transform phlegm and expel wind:
- Wind-phlegm obstructing the channels with facial paralysis.
  *+ Bai Jiang Can, Quan Xie*
- Tetanus. *+ Tian Ma, Fang Feng*
- Migraine headache. *+ Bai Zhi, Chuan Xiong*

### 2. For scrofula or subcutaneous nodules due to accumulation of phlegm, and snakebite, apply topically to relieve toxicity and dissipate nodules.

[Dosage] 3-6 g. Process before oral administration.

[Precautions] Contraindicated during pregnancy.

# Bai Jie Zi

*Semen Sinapis*
*Acrid, warm; Lung*

[Characteristics] Bai Jie Zi has the functions of dispersing and moving. It specifically acts on the interstitial layer between the skin and muscles to effectively resolve phlegm. It is used for phlegm obstructing the flow of qi with coughing and wheezing, and phlegm obstructing the channels with numbness of the limbs.

**FUNCTIONS • INDICATIONS & MAJOR COMBINATIONS**

### 1. Transform phlegm and regulate the qi:
- Phlegm obstruction and qi stagnation with cough, copious sputum, stifling sensation in the chest and poor appetite. *+ Su Zi, Lai Fu Zi*

### 2. Dissipate nodules and unblock the collaterals:
- Damp-phlegm obstructing the meridians and collaterals with joint pain, numbness of the limbs or yin type of gangrene with discharge.

[Dosage] 3-10 g. Mix the powder with vinegar and apply topically.

[Comments] Currently, it is used to treat pleurisy and reduce pleural effusion.

# Jie Geng

*Radix Platycodonis*
*Bitter, acrid, neutral; Lung*

[**Characteristics**] It mainly enters the Lung channel. Characterized by its ability to open up and to disperse Lung qi, it can expel phlegm, stop coughing and benefit the throat. Neutral in nature, it can be applied in either heat or cold conditions of coughing with copious sputum. Moreover, it disperses Lung qi, promotes the discharge of pus, and can be used to treat Lung abscess. Jie Geng, a guiding herb, light and floating, guides other herbs to the Lung channel.

| FUNCTIONS • INDICATIONS & MAJOR COMBINATIONS |
|---|
| **1. Disperse Lung qi and stop coughing:**<br>• Coughing with copious sputum and focal distention of the chest and diaphragm.<br>— Wind-cold. *+ Zi Su Ye, Xing Ren*<br>— Wind-heat. *+ Sang Ye, Xing Ren*<br>— Qi stagnation and phlegm obstruction. *+ Zhi Qiao, Gua Lou Pi* |
| **2. Benefit the throat:**   w/ Gan Cao = Jie Geng Gan Cao Tang<br>• Exterior wind-heat condition with cough, sore throat and loss of voice. *+ Niu Bang Zi, Chan Tui* |
| **3. Expel phlegm and promote the discharge of pus:**<br>• Lung abscess with chest pain, coughing up purulent and bloody sputum. *+ Lu Gen, Yu Xing Cao* |
| **4. The effect of floating helps guide other herbs up to the Lung.** |

[**Dosage**] 3-10 g.

[**Precautions**] It is not recommended for conditions of rebellious qi with vomiting, hiccup and dizziness or hemoptysis due to yin deficiency with empty fire.

[**Comments**] ❶ Jie Geng is light weight and has an ascending effect; it can assist in carrying other herbs in the prescription upward to the Lung. Jie Geng is commonly prescribed for upper burner disorders, especially for those of the chest, diaphragm and throat, known as the carrier of the prescription.

❷ Among the organs metabolizing water, the Lung functions to regulate water passages at the upper burner. When Lung qi fails to disperse and metabolize water, edema occurs. To treat edema, Jie Geng is added to the prescription because it opens up and disperses Lung qi. This effect is described as "open the lid of the tea pot to facilitate the surge of water flow."

**Herbs that Warm and Transform Cold-Phlegm**

# Xuan Fu Hua

*Flos Inulae*
*Bitter, acrid, salty, slightly warm; Lung, Stomach, Spleen*

[Characteristics] Characterized by its effects of redirecting the rebellious qi and expelling phlegm, it is a common herb for phlegm obstruction and qi stagnation resulting in coughing and wheezing with copious sputum, and phlegm-dampness obstructing in the middle burner with vomiting and focal distention.

**FUNCTIONS • INDICATIONS & MAJOR COMBINATIONS**

**1. Redirect the qi down and expel phlegm:**
- Cold-phlegm with coughing and wheezing. *+ Sheng Jiang, Ban Xia*
- Phlegm-heat with coughing and wheezing. *+ Jie Geng, Sang Bai Pi*

**2. Descend the rebellious qi and stop vomiting:**
- Spleen and Stomach qi deficiency and phlegm-dampness rebelling upwards with nausea, vomiting and focal distention in the epigastrium. *+ Ban Xia, Dai Zhe Shi*

[Dosage] 3-10 g. Place into the mesh bags before decoction.

[Comments] There is an ancient proverb, "all flowers float and ascend; Xuan Fu Hua, however, is the flower that descends."

# Bai Qian

*Rhizoma Cynanchi Stauntonii*
*Acrid, sweet, slightly warm; Lung*

[Characteristics] Expels phlegm and redirects rebellious qi downward; Bai Qian is used when Lung qi fails to disperse causing wheezing and coughing up copious sputum regardless of cold or heat patterns.

**FUNCTIONS • INDICATIONS & MAJOR COMBINATIONS**

**Expel phlegm, redirect the qi downward and stop coughing:**
- Stagnation and blockage of Lung qi with wheezing and coughing up copious sputum.
  — Due to cold. *+ Ban Xia, Zi Wan*
  — Due to heat. *+ Sang Bai Pi, Di Gu Pi*
- Exterior wind-cold with cough. *+ Jing Jie, Jie Geng*

[Dosage] 3-10 g.

# Gua Lou

*Fructus Trichosanthis*
*Sweet, cold; Lung, Stomach, Large Intestine*

[Characteristics] Acts on the upper burner to clear Lung heat, transform phlegm and stop coughing; acts on the lower burner to clear heat, moisten the intestines and unblock the obstruction of bowel movements; it also expands the middle burner and facilitates the flow of qi, and dissipates the nodules. It is commonly used for cough due to phlegm-heat, dry cough related to Lung dryness, Chest Painful Obstruction, and constipation due to intestinal dryness. It can also treat abscesses.

| FUNCTIONS • INDICATIONS & MAJOR COMBINATIONS |
|---|
| **1. Clear the Lung and transform phlegm:** |
|     • Lung-heat with coughing up yellow sticky sputum. *+ Zhe Bei Mu, Zhi Mu* |
|     • Phlegm-heat accumulation with yellow sticky sputum and stifling sensation in the chest. *+ Huang Qin, Dan Nan Xing* |
| **2. Expand the chest and facilitate the flow of qi:** |
|     • Chest Painful Obstruction due to cold-phlegm obstructing the movement of yang qi. *+ Xie Bai, Ban Xia* |
|     • Phlegm-heat accumulation with focal distention in the chest and epigastrium, and pain upon palpation. *+ Ban Xia, Huang Lian* |
| **3. Moisten the intestines and unblock the obstruction of bowel movements:** |
|     • Intestinal dryness with constipation. *+ Huo Ma Ren, Yu Li Ren* |
| **4. Breast abscess with swelling and pain or Lung abscess with purulent and bloody sputum.** |

[Dosage] 10-30 g.

[Precautions] Incompatible with Wu Tou.

[Comments] ❶ The alternative name is Quan Gua Lou.

❷ Quan Gua Lou is the entire fruit, while the peel and seeds are used as herbs. The root of the plant is also an herb. The differentiations are:

**Gua Lou Ren** mainly moistens the Lung to transform phlegm, and moistens the intestines to unblock the obstruction of bowel movements. 10-15 g.

**Gou Lou Pi** primarily clears Lung heat, transforms phlegm, facilitates the flow of qi and expands the chest. 6-10 g.

**Gou Lou Gen**, also known as Tian Hua Fen, is categorized into the herbs that clear heat and drain fire.

# Bei Mu

*Bulbus Fritillariae Cirrhosae/ Bulbus Fritillariae Thunbergii*
*Bitter, sweet, slightly cold/ Bitter, cold; Lung, Heart*

[Characteristics] Bei Mu includes Chuan Bei Mu and Zhe Bei Mu; both transform phlegm, stop coughing, clear heat and dissipate nodules. Chuan Bei Mu is bitter, sweet and slightly cold in nature; the sweet property helps moisten the Lung for dry cough due to Lung dryness, and chronic cough due to Lung deficiency. Zhe Bei Mu is bitter and cold to drain fire and clear heat for exterior condition with cough, phlegm-heat with coughing and wheezing, and sores, abscesses and scrofula.

**FUNCTIONS • INDICATIONS & MAJOR COMBINATIONS**

### 1. Transform phlegm and stop coughing:
- Phlegm-heat with cough. *+ Zhi Mu*
- Lung deficiency with chronic cough, scanty sputum and dry throat, use Chuan Bei Mu *+ Sha Shen, Mai Men Dong*
- Exterior wind-heat or phlegm-fire accumulation with cough, use Zhe Bei Mu *+ Sang Ye, Niu Bang Zi*

### 2. Clear heat and dissipate nodules: (Mostly use Zhe Bei Mu)
- Scrofula. *+ Xuan Shen, Mu Li*
- Sores, carbuncles or breast abscess. *+ Pu Gong Ying, Lian Qiao*
- Lung abscess. *+ Yu Xing Cao, Lu Gen*
- Goiter. *+Xia Ku Cao, Kun Bu*

[Dosage] 3-10 g. 1-1.5 g for powder form.

[Precautions] Incompatible with Wu Tou.

# Zhu Ru

*Caulis Bambusae in Taenia*
*Sweet, slightly cold; Lung, Stomach, Gallbladder*

[Characteristics] It primarily clears Lung heat to transform phlegm and clears Stomach heat to stop vomiting. It also eliminates irritability and quiets the mind. Zhu Ru is used for phlegm-heat with cough, Stomach heat with vomiting, and phlegm-heat with irritability.

| FUNCTIONS • INDICATIONS & MAJOR COMBINATIONS |
| --- |
| **1. Clear heat and transform phlegm:** |
| • Lung heat with yellow sticky sputum. *+ Huang Qin, Gua Lou* |
| • Phlegm-heat disturbing upward with stifling sensation in the chest, copious sputum, irritability, insomnia, agitation, palpitation and bitter taste in the mouth. *+ Ban Xia, Zhi Shi* |
| **2. Clear heat and stop vomiting:** |
| • Stomach deficient heat with vomiting. *+ Chen Pi, Ren Shen* |
| • Phlegm-heat accumulation with irritability, focal distention and vomiting. *+ Huang Lian, Chen Pi* |

[Dosage] 6-10 g. Ginger-fried form is often used to treat vomiting.

# Qian Hu

*Radix Peucedani*
*Bitter, acrid, slightly cold; Lung*

[Characteristics] Descends the qi, transforms phlegm and stops coughing, as well as disperses wind-heat; therefore, it is especially useful for phlegm-heat cough accompanied by exterior condition.

| FUNCTIONS • INDICATIONS & MAJOR COMBINATIONS |
| --- |
| **1. Redirect the qi down and transform phlegm:** |
| • Lung qi unable to descend with wheezing and coughing up sticky sputum. *+ Sang Bai Pi, Xing Ren* |
| **2. Disperse wind-heat:** |
| • Exterior wind-heat with fever, aversion to wind, cough and sore throat. *+ Niu Bang Zi, Sang Ye* |

[Dosage] 6- 10 g.

**Herbs that Clear and Transform Phlegm-Heat**

# Hai Zao

*Sargassum*
*Salty, cold; Liver, Kidney, Stomach*

**[Characteristics]** Salty and cold in nature, Hai Zao mainly transforms phlegm, softens hardness and dissipates nodules. It is the primary herb for goiter and scrofula due to phlegm-fire complex.

**FUNCTIONS • INDICATIONS & MAJOR COMBINATIONS**

**1. Resolve phlegm and soften hardness:**
- Goiter. *+ Kun Bu, Bei Mu*
- Scrofula. *+ Xia Ku Cao, Xuan Shen*
- Swollen and painful testicles. *+ Ju He, Kun Bu*

**2. Promote urination and reduce edema.**

**[Dosage]** 10-15 g.

**[Precautions]** Incompatible with Gan Cao. However, recent clinical reports indicate that the combination of Hai Zao and Gan Cao is safe.

# Kun Bu

*Thallus Laminariae seu Eckloniae*
*Salty, cold; Liver, Kidney, Stomach*

**[Characteristics]** Has similar but stronger effects than Hai Zao, Kun Bu is commonly combined with Hai Zao as mutual reinforcement for goiter and scrofula.

**FUNCTIONS • INDICATIONS & MAJOR COMBINATIONS**

**1. Resolve phlegm and soften hardness:**
- Goiter and scrofula. *+ Hai Zao, Bei Mu*
- Swollen and painful testicles. *+ Ju He, Hai Zao*

**2. Promote urination and reduce edema when used with diuretic herbs.**

**[Dosage]** 10-15 g.

# Xing Ren

*Semen Armeniacae Amarum*
*Bitter, slightly warm, slightly toxic; Lung, Large Intestine*

[Characteristics] Enters the Lung and Large Intestine channels; it is bitter to descend the qi and helps stop coughing and calm wheezing. Xing Ren is indicated for coughing and wheezing regardless of how it was acquired, whether by exterior attacks or internal injuries, cold or heat, deficiency or excess. It is warm, therefore, appropriate for exterior wind-cold attacking the Lung with productive cough and copious sputum. In addition, Xing Ren contains rich oil and can be used to treat constipation due to dryness of the intestines.

| FUNCTIONS • INDICATIONS & MAJOR COMBINATIONS |
|---|
| **1. Stop coughing and calm wheezing:** |
| • Patterns of coughing and wheezing. |
| — Exterior wind-cold attacking the Lung. *+ Ma Huang, Gan Cao* |
| — Exterior wind-heat attacking the Lung. *+ Sang Ye, Ju Hua* |
| — Warm-dryness attacking the Lung. *+ Sang Ye, Bei Mu* |
| — Heat accumulated in the Lung. *+ Ma Huang, Shi Gao* |
| **2. Moisten the intestines and unblock the obstruction of bowel movements:** |
| • Constipation due to intestinal dryness. *+ Huo Ma Ren, Dang Gui* |

[Dosage] 3-10 g. Add into the decoction towards the end.

[Precautions] Slightly toxic, do not exceed the recommended dosage. Use with caution in infants.

[Comments] ❶ Xing Ren includes Ku Xing Ren and Tian Xing Ren:

**Ku Xing Ren**, which is bitter and draining in nature, descends the qi and effectively stops coughing and calms wheezing, especially for exterior conditions. It is slightly toxic.

**Tian Xing Ren**, sweet and neutral, is used as a supplement to nourish and moisten the Lung to stop dry cough.

❷ Both Xing Ren and Ma Huang enter the Lung channel; together as mutual assistance, they enhance their effects to treat coughing and wheezing due to exterior wind-cold attacking the Lung. Ma Huang tends to dispel wind-cold and disperse Lung qi; Xing Ren tends to descend Lung qi. One disperses and the other descends, together they restore the function of Lung qi; consequently, coughing and wheezing are resolved.

**Herbs that Stop Coughing and Calm Wheezing**

# Bai Bu

### Radix Stemonae
### *Sweet, bitter, slightly warm; Lung*

[Characteristics] Bai Bu is neutral and mainly enters the Lung channel. It moistens the Lung and descends the qi to stop cough. It is widely used for cough, especially for chronic and deficient types, as an important herb for Lung consumption with cough. In addition, it also eradicates parasites.

**FUNCTIONS • INDICATIONS & MAJOR COMBINATIONS**

### 1. Moisten the Lung and stop coughing:
- Exterior wind-cold with cough. *+ Jie Geng, Zi Wan*
- Children with whooping cough. *+ Sha Shen, Chuan Bei Mu*
- Lung consumption with cough. *+ Mai Men Dong, Sheng Di Huang*

### 2. Expel parasites and kill lice:
- For head or body lice, use the decoction as an external wash.
- For pinworms, the decoction is used as an enema.

[Dosage] 6-10 g. Honey-fried form is used for chronic or deficiency cough.

# Zi Wan

### Radix Asteris
### *Bitter, sweet, slightly warm; Lung*

[Characteristics] Moistens the Lung and descends Lung qi, stops coughing and calms wheezing. Zi Wan is slightly warm; with the appropriate combinations, it can be used for all patterns of coughing and wheezing.

**FUNCTIONS • INDICATIONS & MAJOR COMBINATIONS**

### Moisten the Lung, descend Lung qi and stop coughing:
- Exterior condition with cough and itchiness of the throat. *+ Jing Jie, Bai Qian*
- Lung deficiency with chronic cough and hemoptysis. *+ Zhi Mu, Kuan Dong Hua*

[Dosage] 6-10 g. Raw form is used for exterior condition with cough, while honey-fried form is used for Lung deficiency with chronic cough.

# Kuan Dong Hua

*Flos Farfarae*
*Acrid, warm; Lung*

[Characteristics] This is an important herb for productive cough. It has similar effects as Zi Wan in moistening the Lung and descending Lung qi. These two herbs are usually combined together for mutual reinforcement in all types of coughing and wheezing.

| FUNCTIONS • INDICATIONS & MAJOR COMBINATIONS |
|---|
| **Moisten the Lung, descend Lung qi and stop coughing:**<br>• Exterior condition with cough. *+ Jing Jie, Bai Qian*<br>• Chronic cough with blood-tinged sputum. *+ Zi Wan, Zhi Mu*<br>• Phlegm-heat with cough. *+ Sang Bai Pi, Xing Ren*<br>• Cold in the Lung with wheezing and coughing up copious sputum. *+ Zi Wan, Ma Huang* |

[Dosage] 6-10 g. Use the raw or honey-fried form.

# Su Zi

*Fructus Perillae*
*Acrid, warm; Lung, Large Intestine*

[Characteristics] It enters the Lung channel to descend Lung qi and resolve phlegm obstruction and qi stagnation with coughing, wheezing and stifling sensation in the chest; it enters the Large Intestine channel to moisten the intestines and unblock the obstruction of bowel movements.

| FUNCTIONS • INDICATIONS & MAJOR COMBINATIONS |
|---|
| **1. Descend Lung qi, stop coughing and calm wheezing:**<br>• Phlegm obstruction and qi stagnation with coughing up copious sputum, stifling sensation in the chest and lack of appetite. *+ Bai Jie Zi, Lai Fu Zi*<br>• Coughing and wheezing with abundant watery sputum, stifling sensation of the chest and diaphragm. *+ Hou Po, Ban Xia* |
| **2. Moisten the intestines and unblock the obstruction of bowel movements:**<br>• Constipation due to intestinal dryness. *+ Huo Ma Ren, Gua Lou Ren* |

[Dosage] 6-10 g.

# Sang Bai Pi

*Cortex Mori*
*Sweet, cold; Lung*

[Characteristics] It exclusively enters the Lung channel and drains Lung heat to calm coughing and wheezing. Also San Bai Pi drains Lung excess to resolve phlegm and facilitate the drainage of water retention. It is especially effective in treating Lung heat and phlegm-fire complex with coughing and wheezing.

**FUNCTIONS • INDICATIONS & MAJOR COMBINATIONS**

**1. Drain heat from the Lung and calm wheezing:**
   - Lung heat with coughing, wheezing and copious sputum. *+ Di Gu Pi, Gan Cao*

**2. Promote urination and reduce swelling:**
   - *Pi Shui* due to excessive dampness and Spleen deficiency. *+ Da Fu Pi, Fu Ling Pi*

[Dosage] 10-15 g. Raw form is used for draining Lung excess and promoting urination; honey-fried form is used for Lung deficiency.

# Pi Pa Ye

*Folium Eriobotryae*
*Bitter, cool; Lung, Stomach*

[Characteristics] Bitter and cool, Pi Pa Ye mainly enters the Lung and Stomach channels. It clears Lung heat to calm coughing and resolve phlegm, as well as clears Stomach heat to redirect rebellious qi downward and to stop vomiting.

**FUNCTIONS • INDICATIONS & MAJOR COMBINATIONS**

**1. Transform phlegm and stop coughing:**
   - Wind-heat with cough. *+ Qian Hu, Sang Ye*
   - Dry-heat with cough. *+ Sang Bai Pi, Sha Shen*
   - Lung deficiency with chronic cough. *+ E Jiao, Bai He*

**2. Redirect rebellious qi and stop vomiting:**
   - Stomach heat with thirst, hiccup, nausea and vomiting. *+ Zhu Ru*

[Dosage] 10-15 g. Honey-fried form is recommended for cough, and the raw form is recommended for vomiting.

# Ting Li Zi

*Semen Lepidii seu Descurainiae*
*Bitter, acrid, very cold; Lung, Bladder*

[Characteristics] Drains Lung excess to resolve phlegm and facilitate the drainage of water retention. It is used for stagnation and blockage of Lung qi causing congested fluids with wheezing and stifling sensation in the chest limiting the patient from lying down, or for water retention in the chest and abdominal cavities.

| FUNCTIONS • INDICATIONS & MAJOR COMBINATIONS |
|---|
| **1. Drain the water retention from the Lung and calm wheezing:**<br>• Excessive phlegm with coughing, wheezing, unable to lie down flat and systemic edema. *+ Da Zao* |
| **2. Promote urination and reduce edema:**<br>• Excess patterns of water retention in the chest and abdominal cavities with edema and dysuria. *+ Fang Ji, Da Huang* |

[Dosage] 3-10 g.

[Comments] Currently, it treats exudative pleurisy with pleural effusion.


# Ma Dou Ling

*Fructus Aristolochiae*
*Bitter, slightly acrid, cold; Lung, Large Intestine*

[Characteristics] Clears and descends Lung qi with its cold nature. Ma Dou Ling can be used for productive cough and wheezing of heat type.

| FUNCTIONS • INDICATIONS & MAJOR COMBINATIONS |
|---|
| **1. Clear heat from the Lung, transform phlegm and stop coughing:**<br>• Lung heat with productive cough. *+ Sang Bai Pi, Huang Qin*<br>• Lung deficient heat with coughing and wheezing. *+ Xing Ren, Niu Bang Zi*<br>• Yin deficiency and empty fire with coughing up blood-tinged sputum. *+ E Jiao, Bai Ji* |
| **2. Hemorrhaging from swollen painful hemorrhoids.** |

[Dosage] 3-10 g. This herb may induce vomiting; therefore, it is not recommended to exceed the regular dose range.

## [Remarks & Differentiations]

**Ban Xia and Tian Nan Xing:**
> Common herbs that warm and transform cold-phlegm.

**Bei Mu and Gua Lou:**
> Common herbs that clear and transform phlegm-heat.

**Xing Ren and Su Zi:**
> Common herbs that stop coughing and calm wheezing.

Coughing and wheezing are often accompanied by phlegm, as excessive phlegm causes coughing and wheezing. Herbs that transform phlegm usually have additional effect in calming coughing and wheezing, and the majority of herbs that stop coughing and calm wheezing can transform phlegm. Therefore, in clinical application, there is no definite distinction between these herbs.

### Ban Xia — Tian Nan Xing

|   | Ban Xia | Tian Nan Xing |
|---|---------|---------------|
| C | Dry dampness and transform phlegm. Apply topically to reduce swelling and dissipate nodules. | |
| D | • Primarily used for phlegm-dampness.<br><br>• Descends the rebellious qi and stops vomiting.<br>• Reduces focal distention. | • Extremely toxic, warm and drying, mainly used for wind-phlegm, also used for stubborn cough with sputum. |

### Tian Nan Xing — Dan Nan Xing

|   | Tian Nan Xing | Dan Nan Xing |
|---|---------------|--------------|
| C | Transform phlegm. | |
| D | • Bitter, warm and extremely drying to dry dampness, transform phlegm, dispel wind-phlegm and alleviate tremors. | • Bitter, cool and moist in nature to clear heat, transform phlegm and alleviate convulsions. |

## Bai Fu Zi — Bai Jie Zi

|   | Bai Fu Zi | Bai Jie Zi |
|---|---|---|
| C | Dry dampness and transform phlegm. ||
| D | • Effectively dispels wind-phlegm from the head region. | • Resolves damp-phlegm obstructed in the meridians and collaterals.<br>• Benefits the flow of qi. |

## Ban Xia — Bei Mu

|   | Ban Xia | Bei Mu |
|---|---|---|
| C | Transform phlegm and stop coughing. ||
| D | • Acrid, warm to dry dampness and transform phlegm for damp-phlegm and cold-phlegm.<br>• Reduces focal distention and dissipates nodules for fullness in the chest and epigastrium. | • Sweet, cold to clear heat, moisten the dryness and transform phlegm for phlegm-heat and dry-phlegm.<br>• Clears heat and dissipates nodules for goiter and scrofula. |

## Xing Ren — Jie Geng

|   | Xing Ren | Jie Geng |
|---|---|---|
| C | Disseminate and open up Lung qi, stop coughing and calm wheezing. Mostly combined for mutual reinforcement. ||
| D | • Descends Lung qi.<br>• Moistens the intestines and unblocks the obstruction of bowel movements. | • Primarily ascends to disperse Lung qi, and transform phlegm. |

## Xing Ren — Su Zi

|   | Xing Ren | Su Zi |
|---|---|---|
| C | Enter the Lung to descend Lung qi, stop coughing and calm wheezing. Enter the Large Intestine to moisten the intestines and unblock the bowel. ||
| D | • Indicated for coughing and wheezing caused by exterior attacks or internal injuries, cold or heat, deficiency or excess. | • Commonly used for coughing and wheezing with abundant watery sputum, stifling sensation of the chest and diaphragm. |

**Herbs that Transform Phlegm and Stop Coughing**

## Xing Ren — Qian Hu

| | Xing Ren | Qian Hu |
|---|---|---|
| C | Descend qi, transform phlegm and stop coughing. ||
| D | • Warm in nature, used for exterior wind-cold attacking the Lung with productive cough and wheezing. | • Slightly cold, especially effective for phlegm-heat cough accompanied by exterior conditions. |

## Sang Bai Pi — Ting Li Zi

| | Sang Bai Pi | Ting Li Zi |
|---|---|---|
| C | Drain pathogenic factors from the Lung and calm wheezing. Promote urination and reduce swelling. ||
| D | • Drains heat from the Lung.<br><br>• Less potent in promoting urination, used for mild conditions of edema, such as *Pi Shui*. | • Drains the stagnation and blockage of Lung qi.<br>• Strongly promotes urination for severe cases of edema, such as water retention in the chest or abdominal cavities. |

## Zi Wan — Bai Bu — Kuan Dong Hua

| | Zi Wan | Bai Bu | Kuan Dong Hua |
|---|---|---|---|
| C | Exclusively enter the Lung channel. Moisten the Lung, descend qi, transform phlegm and stop coughing. Commonly combined for mutual reinforcement to treat all patterns of cough, especially effective for chronic and deficient types. |||
| D | • Strongly transforms phlegm. | • Relatively stronger to stop coughing.<br>• Expels parasites and kills lice. | • Relatively stronger to stop coughing. |

# HERBS THAT
## Relieve Food Stagnation 8

With this group of herbs, the main functions are to improve digestion and relieve food stagnation. When relieving food retention, herbs from this group also strengthen the Spleen, improve appetite and harmonize the middle burner. They are used to treat retention of food with focal distention and fullness in the epigastrium and abdomen, lack of appetite, nausea, vomiting and irregular bowel movements.

Food stagnation can obstruct the flow of qi and cause Spleen and Stomach qi stagnation; therefore, these herbs are commonly combined with herbs that regulate the qi. When food stagnation is accompanied with excessive dampness, add herbs that transform dampness and revive the Spleen. When food stagnation is accompanied with constipation, herbs that drain downward are added. When food stagnation is due to Spleen and Stomach deficiency, the treatment principle should be modified to strengthen the function of the middle burner. This in turn would likely take care of the stagnation.

# Shan Zha

*Fructus Crataegi*
*Sour, sweet, slightly warm; Spleen, Stomach, Liver*

**[Characteristics]** Effective in relieving food stagnation as well as reviving the Spleen and improving the appetite, Shan Zha is especially useful for meat or grease stagnation. It also invigorates blood and dispels stasis.

**FUNCTIONS • INDICATIONS & MAJOR COMBINATIONS**

**1. Relieve food stagnation and resolve accumulations:**
- Retention of meat and greasy diet with distention of the epigastrium and abdomen. *+ Shen Qu, Mai Ya*
- Food retention and indigestion with abdominal pain and diarrhea. Administer the scorched and powdered form.

**2. Invigorate the blood and dispel stasis:**
- Post-partum blood stasis with abdominal pain and lochioschesis. *+ Chuan Xiong, Dang Gui*
- Hernia disorder with distention and pain. *+ Xiao Hui Xiang, Ju He*

**3. Hypertension, coronary arterial disease and hyperlipidemia.**

**[Dosage]** 10-15 g. May increase to 30 g.

# Lai Fu Zi

*Semen Raphani*
*Acrid, sweet, neutral; Spleen, Stomach, Lung*

**[Characteristics]** It relieves food stagnation and reduces distention, as well as descends the flow of qi and transforms phlegm.

**FUNCTIONS • INDICATIONS & MAJOR COMBINATIONS**

**1. Relieve food stagnation and resolve accumulations:**
- Food retention and indigestion with abdominal distention and pain. *+ Shan Zha, Chen Pi*
- Food stagnation accompanied by Spleen qi deficiency. *+ Bai Zhu*

**2. Descend the flow of qi and transform phlegm:**
- Excess type of coughing and wheezing with copious sputum. *+ Bai Jie Zi, Su Zi*

**[Dosage]** 6-10 g.

# Ji Nei Jin

*Endothelium Corneum Gigeriae Galli*
*Sweet, neutral; Spleen, Stomach, Bladder, Small Intestine*

[Characteristics] Of all the herbs that relieve food stagnation, Ji Nei Jin has the strongest effect to relieve all types of food retention. It also strengthens the Spleen and Stomach, as well as astringes and restrains the leakage.

| FUNCTIONS • INDICATIONS & MAJOR COMBINATIONS |
|---|
| **1. Strengthen the Spleen to reduce food stagnation:**<br>  • Food retention and indigestion. *+ Shan Zha, Mai Ya*<br>  • Childhood nutritional impairment accompanied with food retention. *+ Bai Zhu* |
| **2. Bind the essence and restrain the leakage:**<br>  • Spermatorrhea, nocturnal emission and enuresis. |
| **3. For calculi of the urinary and biliary tracts, commonly** *+ Jin Qian Cao* |

[Dosage] 1.5-3 g. Use the raw form to resolve the calculi, and the fried form to strengthen the Spleen and reduce food retention.


# Shen Qu

*Massa Fermentata*
*Sweet, acrid, warm; Spleen, Stomach*

[Characteristics] Weaker in strength to relieve general food stagnation in comparison to Ji Nei Jin, Shen Qu is more effective in resolving food stagnation of grains.

| FUNCTIONS • INDICATIONS & MAJOR COMBINATIONS |
|---|
| **1. Relieve food stagnation and harmonize the Stomach:**<br>  • Food retention and indigestion with distention of the epigastrium and abdomen. *+ Shan Zha, Mai Ya* |
| **2. Use as an excipient for binding other ingredients into pill form.** |

[Dosage] 6-15 g.

[Comments] The scorched herbs of Shen Qu, Shan Zha and Mai Ya are very often combined in clinical practice, known as Jiao San Xian, or three scorched herbs. This is the basic combination for treating food stagnation.

# Mai Ya

*Fructus Hordei Germinatus*
*Sweet, neutral; Spleen, Stomach, Liver*

[Characteristics] Less effective in relieving food stagnation compared to Shen Qu, Mai Ya is especially effective in relieving food retention of wheat. In addition, it inhibits lactation.

**FUNCTIONS • INDICATIONS & MAJOR COMBINATIONS**

**1. Reduce food stagnation and strengthen the Spleen and Stomach:**
  • Food retention and indigestion of wheat. *+ Shan Zha, Shen Qu*

**2. For women who wish to discontinue breastfeeding, decoct the raw herb in large dose.**

[Dosage] 10-15 g. May increase dose to 120 g.

[Precautions] Contraindicated during breastfeeding.

# Gu Ya

*Fructus Setariae Germinatus*
*Sweet, neutral; Spleen, Stomach*

[Characteristics] Of all herbs to relieve food stagnation, Gu Ya is least effective. It is often used to nourish Stomach and relieve stagnation of grains.

**FUNCTIONS • INDICATIONS & MAJOR COMBINATIONS**

**Relieve food stagnation and harmonize the middle burner:**
  • Patterns of food stagnation and Spleen deficiency with poor appetite.
    — Severe food stagnation. *+ Mai Ya, Shen Qu*
    — Severe Spleen deficiency. *+ Dang Shen, Bai Zhu*

[Dosage] 10-15 g. May increase the dose to 30 g.

## [Remarks & Differentiations]

Depending on the various types of food consumed, food stagnation can be caused by a heavy diet consisting of meat, grease, grains, and/or wheat. Herbs that relieve food stagnation are distinctive for various conditions of food stagnation because of their individual therapeutic effects.

Herbs in this category have a way of strengthening the Spleen, harmonizing the Stomach and regulating the middle burner, in addition to its primary function of relieving food stagnation. Herbs that have stronger effects in relieving food stagnation have relatively weaker strength in harmonizing the Stomach; in contrary, herbs that are more effective in harmonizing the Stomach are relatively mild in relieving food stagnation.

**Herbs that Relieve Food Stagnation**

# HERBS THAT
## Regulate the Qi 9

Herbs in this chapter direct the qi to flow smoothly. Most of these herbs are aromatic and warm, and are either acrid or bitter to migrate or descend. They enter the Liver and Stomach channels, and functions to regulate the qi and strengthen the Spleen, spread constrained Liver qi, move the qi and alleviate pain, break up qi stagnation and dissipate nodules, and redirect rebellious qi downward. Qi regulators are used for qi stagnation of the Spleen and Stomach with distention and fullness in the epigastrium and abdomen, Liver constraint and qi stagnation with pain in the hypochondriac regions and cold hernia disorder with abdominal pain, and for rebellious Stomach qi with hiccups and vomiting.

Herbs that regulate the qi tend to be acrid, dispersing and drying, and they can easily injure the yin and consume the qi; therefore, use with caution.

*Chen Pi*

# Ju Pi

*Pericarpium Citri Reticulatae*
*Acrid, bitter, warm; Spleen, Lung*

[Characteristics] Acrid to promote the qi flow, bitter and warm to dry dampness and phlegm, aromatic to revive the Spleen, Ju Pi is the imperial herb to move the qi, strengthen the Spleen, dry dampness and resolve phlegm for qi stagnation and dampness accumulation in the middle burner, and cough with copious sputum.

**FUNCTIONS • INDICATIONS & MAJOR COMBINATIONS**

### 1. Move the qi and regulate the middle burner:
- Spleen and Stomach qi stagnation with epigastric and abdominal distention and fullness. *+ Zhi Qiao, Mu Xiang*
- Liver invading the Spleen with painful diarrhea. *+ Bai Zhu, Bai Shao*
- Spleen deficiency with qi stagnation. *+ Dang Shen, Bai Zhu*

### 2. Dry dampness and resolve phlegm:
- Phlegm-dampness accumulation in the Lung with copious sputum. *+ Ban Xia, Fu Ling*
- Dampness accumulation in the middle burner with abdominal distention, and thick greasy tongue coating. *+ Cang Zhu, Hou Po*

[Dosage] 3-10 g.

[Comments] ❶ Good quality Ju Pi is usually stored for a long time; therefore, the alternative name is Chen Pi, or aged peel. The best quality Chen Pi is found in the province of Guangdong; therefore, another alternative name is Guang Chen Pi.

❷ Below are herbs from the same plant:

**Ju He** spreads Liver qi, dissipates nodules and alleviates pain. It is primarily used for hernia, testicular distended pain and lumps on the breast.

**Ju Luo** promotes the movement of qi and transforms phlegm. It is primarily used for phlegm obstructing the meridians and collaterals.

**Ju Ye** spreads Liver qi and dissipates nodules. It is primarily used for lumps or abscesses on the breast.

## [Addendum]
## Hua Ju Hong
### *Exocarpium Citri Grandis*
Bitter, acrid and warm, it promotes the movement of qi and transforms phlegm. It is warmer and dryer than Chen Pi; therefore, it is primarily used for coughing with copious sputum and absence of heat signs. 3-10 g.

# Qing Pi

*Pericarpium Citri Reticulatae Viride*
*Bitter, acrid, warm; Liver, Gallbladder, Stomach*

[Characteristics] With similar properties and relatively stronger effects than Ju Pi, Qing Pi enters the Liver and Gallbladder channels to spread Liver qi, break up qi stagnation and reduce accumulations. It is used for conditions of Liver constraint and qi stagnation with chest and hypochondriac distention and pain, and those of accumulation and stagnation in the Stomach and intestines.

**FUNCTIONS • INDICATIONS & MAJOR COMBINATIONS**

### 1. Spread Liver qi and break up qi stagnation:
- Constrained Liver and qi stagnation with hypochondriac distention and pain. *+ Chai Hu, Yu Jin*
- Constrained Liver and qi stagnation with breast distention and pain or lumps. *+ Ju Ye, Xiang Fu*
- Swollen and painful breast abscess. *+ Gua Lou, Jin Yin Hua*
- Cold type of hernia disorder with abdominal pain. *+ Wu Yao, Xiao Hui Xiang*
- Qi stagnation and blood stasis with *Zheng Jia Ji Ju*.* *+ San Leng, E Zhu*

### 2. Dissipate clumps and reduce stagnation:
- Food retention and qi stagnation. *+ Shan Zha, Mai Ya*
- Severe food retention and qi stagnation. *+ Zhi Shi, Bing Lang*

[Dosage] 3-10 g. Normally, this herb is fried with vinegar.

[Comments] *Zheng Jia Ji Ju**: Refers to four different disorders characterized by the presence of masses in the abdomen with distention and/or pain. *Zheng* is the substantial mass with fixed location and pain; it is classified into disorders of yin organ and blood level; the primary treatment principle for *Zheng* is to invigorate the blood and expel blood stasis. *Jia* is the insubstantial mass with migrating location and pain; it is classified into disorders of yang organ and qi level; the primary treatment principle for *Jia* is to regulate the qi and dissipate the clumps. *Ji* is similar to *Zheng* while *Ju* is similar to *Jia*. In general, these disorders are severe cases of qi stagnation and blood stasis; therefore, strong herbs that break up qi stagnation and/or blood stasis are used to treat these disorders, and these strong herbs are used only for those with sufficient righteous qi.

# Zhi Shi

*Fructus Aurantii Immaturus*
*Bitter, acrid, slightly cold; Spleen, Stomach, Large Intestine*

[Characteristics] Descends downward, Zhi Shi specifically breaks up the stagnant qi in the Stomach and intestines to reduce clumps and resolve focal distention. It also benefits the flow of qi to transform phlegm, and is used for focal distention and fullness in the chest and epigastrium.

**FUNCTIONS • INDICATIONS & MAJOR COMBINATIONS**

### 1. Break up stagnant qi and reduce clumps:
- Heat accumulation with constipation, abdominal distention and pain.
  *+ Da Huang, Hou Po*
- Food retention and indigestion with epigastric and abdominal distention and fullness. *+ Shan Zha, Shen Qu*
- Spleen deficiency and qi stagnation. *+ Bai Zhu*
- Damp-heat dysentery with tenesmus. *+ Da Huang, Huang Lian*

### 2. Transform phlegm and expel focal distention:
- Chest Painful Obstruction due to phlegm-qi complex that obstructs the flow of Heart yang. *+ Xie Bai, Gui Zhi*
- Phlegm-heat disturbing upward with stifling sensation in the chest, palpitation, bitter taste in the mouth and insomnia. *+ Ban Xia, Zhu Ru*

### 3. For prolapse of organs (i.e. rectum, uterus, etc.), combine with herbs that tonify the qi.

[Dosage] 3-10 g.

[Precautions] Use with caution during pregnancy.

[Addendum]
## Zhi Qiao (Zhi Ke)
*Fructus Aurantii*

Zhi Qiao has the same properties and effects, enters the same channels, and has the same dose range as Zhi Shi; however, Zhi Qiao has milder effect. It can effectively promote the movement of qi, expand the middle burner and reduce distention; it is primarily used for the condition of qi stagnation with distention and fullness in the epigastrium and abdomen.

# Xiang Fu

*Rhizoma Cyperi*
*Acrid, slightly bitter, slightly sweet, neutral; Liver, Triple Burner*

[Characteristics] Mainly enters the Liver channel, it spreads Liver qi in patterns of Liver constraint. Moreover, Xiang Fu is commonly used for gynecological disorders and is the imperial herb to regulate menstruation and alleviate pain.

| FUNCTIONS • INDICATIONS & MAJOR COMBINATIONS |
|---|
| **1. Spread and regulate Liver qi:** |
| • Constrained Liver qi with hypochondriac distention and pain. *+ Chai Hu, Bai Shao* |
| • Constrained Liver qi invading the Stomach. *+ Mu Xiang* |
| • Cold type of hernia disorder with abdominal pain. *+ Wu Yao, Xiao Hui Xiang* |
| **2. Promote the movement of qi and alleviate pain:** |
| • Cold congealing and qi stagnation with pain in the epigastric region. *+ Gao Liang Jiang* |
| **3. Regulate menstruation and alleviate pain:** |
| • Constrained Liver qi with irregular menstruation and dysmenorrhea. *+ Dang Gui, Bai Shao* |
| • Constrained Liver qi with breast distention and pain. *+ Chai Hu, Ju Ye* |

[Dosage] 6-10 g.

[Comments] ❶ Xiang Fu is one of two imperial herbs that regulate menstruation and alleviate pain; the other is Dang Gui. For differentiation and application (p. 218).

❷ Xiang Fu is neutral in temperature without having either hot or cold tendencies. In addition to its acrid nature, it is a strong aromatic. With proper combinations, it can be used for qi stagnations of any organs. Moreover, it mainly enters the Liver channel to spread constrained Liver qi. Based on the principle that the circulation of blood follows the movement of qi, it is a common herb for disorders related to menstruation, pregnancy and labor due to Liver qi stagnation. Therefore, this herb has been illustrated as "the general commander for qi stagnation and the chief officer for gynecological disorders".

# Mu Xiang

*Radix Aucklandiae*

*Acrid, bitter, warm; Spleen, Stomach, Gallbladder, Large Intestine*

[Characteristics] Acrid and warm, it moves and disperses. Aromatic in nature, it revives the Spleen. Mu Xiang effectively promotes the movement of qi in the Stomach and intestines to reduce distention and alleviate pain. It is primarily used for distention and fullness in the epigastrium and abdomen and damp-heat dysentery; it is also commonly combined with qi tonics to prevent qi stagnation.

### FUNCTIONS • INDICATIONS & MAJOR COMBINATIONS

#### 1. Promote the movement of qi and alleviate pain:

- Qi stagnation in the Stomach and intestines with epigastric and abdominal distention and pain. *+ Zhi Qiao*
- Damp-heat dysentery. *+ Huang Lian*
- Food retention and qi stagnation with abdominal pain and diarrhea. *+ Bing Lang, Da Huang*
- Damp-heat jaundice. *+ Yu Jin, Yin Chen Hao*

#### 2. Promote the movement of qi and harmonize the middle burner:

- Spleen and Stomach qi deficiency and qi stagnation with abdominal distention and diarrhea. *+ Dang Shen, Sha Ren*

[Dosage] 3-10 g. Raw form is used to move the qi; roasted form stops diarrhea.

[Precautions] Contraindicated in yin deficiency with heat signs.

# Wu Yao

*Radix Linderae*
*Acrid, warm; Lung, Spleen, Kidney, Bladder*

[Characteristics] A warm herb that promotes the movement of qi, Wu Yao facilitates the qi movement of the upper, middle and lower burners to disperse cold and alleviate pain with good effects. It is commonly used for patterns of pain due to cold congealing and qi stagnation.

FUNCTIONS • INDICATIONS & MAJOR COMBINATIONS

**1. Promote the movement of qi, expel cold and alleviate pain:**
- All pain types from cold congealing and qi stagnation.
  — Hypochondriac pain. *+ Xie Bai, Yu Jin*
  — Hernia disorder with abdominal pain. *+ Xiao Hui Xiang*
  — Epigastric and abdominal distended pain. *+ Mu Xiang, Zhi Qiao*

**2. Warm the Kidney and expel cold:**
- Lower burner deficient cold with enuresis. *+ Yi Zhi Ren, Shan Yao*

[Dosage] 3-10 g.
[Comments] The alternative name is Tai Wu Yao.


# Chuan Lian Zi

*Fructus Toosendan*
*Bitter, cold, slightly toxic; Liver, Small Intestine, Bladder*

[Characteristics] Mainly enters the Liver channel, it effectively spreads Liver qi and alleviates pain. As a bitter and cold herb, Chuan Lian Zi is often used in Liver constraint with heat signs. It can also kill parasites.

FUNCTIONS • INDICATIONS & MAJOR COMBINATIONS

**1. Promote the movement of qi and alleviate pain:**
- Constrained Liver qi with heat signs. *+ Yan Hu Suo*
- Cold type of hernia disorder. *+ Xiao Hui Xiang, Wu Zhu Yu*

**2. Kill the parasites for parasites accumulation with abdominal pain.**

[Dosage] 3-10 g.
[Precautions] Not recommended for Spleen and Stomach deficient cold.
[Comments] The alternative name is Jin Ling Zi.

**Herbs that Regulate the Qi**

# Xie Bai

**Bulbus Allii Macrostemonis**
*Acrid, bitter, warm; Lung, Stomach, Large Intestine*

[Characteristics] Acts upward, it unblocks the obstruction of yang qi in the chest and disperses congealed cold. It is the primary herb for Chest Painful Obstruction. Acts downward, it promotes the movement of qi in the Large Intestine.

**FUNCTIONS • INDICATIONS & MAJOR COMBINATIONS**

**1. Unblock the obstruction of yang qi and dissipate clumps:**
- Chest Painful Obstruction due to inactive Heart yang together with phlegm-cold obstruction. *+ Gua Lou*

**2. Promote the movement of qi and guide out the accumulations for dysentery disorder with tenesmus.** *+ Zhi Shi, Mu Xiang*

[Dosage] 3-10 g.

[Comments] In the classic formulas that treat Chest Painful Obstruction, the combination of Xie Bai and Gua Lou is included. Dispersing and warming, Xie Bai unblocks and dispels congealed cold; Gua Lou, on the other hand, expands the chest and facilitates the movement of qi to transform phlegm.

# Chen Xiang

**Lignum Aquilariae Resinatum**
*Acrid, bitter, warm; Spleen, Stomach, Kidney*

[Characteristics] Effectively promotes the qi movement, disperses cold and alleviates pain; Chen Xiang also descends rebellious qi of the Lung and Stomach.

**FUNCTIONS • INDICATIONS & MAJOR COMBINATIONS**

**1. Promote the movement of qi and alleviate pain:**
- Cold congealing and qi stagnation with chest and abdominal distention and pain. *+ Wu Yao, Mu Xiang*

**2. Descend rebellious qi and stop vomiting:**
- Stomach cold with vomiting and hiccup. *+ Ding Xiang, Bai Dou Kou*

**3. Kidney unable to grasp the qi with deficient wheezing.**

[Dosage] 1-1.5 g. Take the powdered form with water.

[Precautions] Use with caution in yin deficiency with heat.

## [Remarks & Differentiations]

### Ju Pi — Qing Pi

|   | Ju Pi | Qing Pi |
|---|-------|---------|
| C | Originate from the same plant. Used for distention and pain in the epigastrium and abdomen, food retention and phlegm accumulation. | |
| D | • Gentle in action, light in nature, it ascends and floats.<br>• Primarily enters the Spleen channel to move qi and regulate the middle burner.<br>• Dries dampness and resolves phlegm. | • Agressive in strength, it desends downward.<br>• Mainly enters the Liver and Gallbladder to spread Liver qi and break up qi stagnation.<br>• Dissipates clumps and reduces accumulations. |

### Zhi Shi — Zhi Qiao

|   | Zhi Shi | Zhi Qiao |
|---|---------|----------|
| C | Same origin, the mature one is called Zhi Qiao, the immature one is Zhi Shi. | |
| D | • Strong in action, breaks up qi stagnation and reduces accumulations.<br>• Descends downward, mostly used for unblocking the obstruction of bowel movements. | • Milder in action, promotes the movement of qi and reduces distention.<br>• Expands the middle burner, mostly used for distention and fullness of epigastrium and abdomen. |

### Xiang Fu — Mu Xiang — Wu Yao

|   | Xiang Fu | Mu Xiang | Wu Yao |
|---|----------|----------|--------|
| C | Facilitate the movement of qi and alleviate pain. | | |
| D | • Mainly enters the Liver channel, spreads and regulates Liver qi.<br>• Regulates the menses. | • Effectively promotes the movement of qi in the Stomach and intestines. | • Facilitates the qi movement of the upper, middle and lower burners, as well as disperses cold. |

# HERBS THAT
## Stop Bleeding 10

Herbs from this category stop bleeding, internally or externally. They function as a hemostatic herb in many ways: cool the blood to stop bleeding, astringe to stop bleeding, transform stasis to stop bleeding, and warm the meridians to stop bleeding. They are used to treat subcutaneous and mucosa bleeding, hemoptysis, hematemesis, hematuria, blood in the stool, Gushing and Leaking Syndromes, and hemorrhages associated with traumatic injuries.

To treat bleeding, based on its root and branch, select the corresponding hemostatic herbs and add the appropriate herbs from other categories to enhance the therapeutic effects. For instance, in the case of bleeding due to heat in the blood, add herbs that clear heat and cool the blood; for bleeding due to deficient cold, combine herbs that augment the qi and warm the yang. Do not use hemostatic herbs alone in conditions of heavy bleeding that may cause the qi to collapse. Instead, adopt the strategy of "strongly tonifying the qi to consolidate the collapse".

Improper use of hemostatic herbs may cause blood stasis. For example, using astringent hemostatic herbs in the early stage of bleeding may cause blood stasis and using large doses of hemostatic herbs with cold nature can also lead to stasis.

# Da Ji

*Herba seu Radix Cirsii Japonici*
*Bitter, sweet, cool; Heart, Liver*

[Characteristics] An important hemostatic herb that cools the blood and stops bleeding, it is used for various hemorrhaging disorders due to heat causing reckless movement of the blood. It also relieves toxicity and reduces swelling.

**FUNCTIONS • INDICATIONS & MAJOR COMBINATIONS**

**1. Cool the blood and stop bleeding:**
  • Heat causing the blood to move recklessly with various bleeding disorders including hemoptysis, subcutaneous and mucosa bleeding, and hematuria. *+ Zhi Zi, Ce Bai Ye*

**2. For sores, carbuncles and toxic swelling, apply the juice of fresh Da Ji topically.**

[Dosage] 10-15 g. May increase dose to 30-60 g. when using fresh form.

# Di Yu

*Radix Sanguisorbae*
*Bitter, sour, slightly cold; Liver, Stomach, Large Intestine*

[Characteristics] Cools the blood and stops bleeding. It is primarily used for hemorrhaging in the lower burner due to heat causing reckless movement of the blood with bloody stool, bleeding hemorrhoids, blood-type of dysentery disorder, Gushing and Leaking Syndromes. Moreover, it is an important herb for burn lesions.

**FUNCTIONS • INDICATIONS & MAJOR COMBINATIONS**

**1. Cool the blood and stop bleeding:**
  • Heat causing the blood to move recklessly with bleeding in the lower burner.
    — Bloody stool and bleeding hemorrhoids. *+ Huai Hua*
    — Gushing and Leaking Syndromes. *+ Sheng Di Huang, Pu Huang*
    — Blood-type of dysentery disorder. *+ Huang Lian, Mu Xiang*

**2. Relieve toxicity and promote healing:**
  • For burn lesions and for eczema, mix the powdered form with sesame oil for topical application to reduce the discharge.

[Dosage] 10-15 g.

# Huai Hua

*Flos Sophorae*
*Bitter, slightly cold; Liver, Large Intestine*

[Characteristics] Cools the blood and stops bleeding. It mainly enters the Large Intestine of the lower burner. It is primarily used for hemorrhaging due to heat causing reckless movement of the blood with bloody stool and bleeding hemorrhoids. It can also be used for hemoptysis, subcutaneous and mucosa bleeding.

| FUNCTIONS • INDICATIONS & MAJOR COMBINATIONS |
| --- |
| **1. Cool the blood and stop bleeding:**<br>• Heat causing the blood to move recklessly with hemorrhaging.<br>— Bloody stool and bleeding hemorrhoids. *+ Di Yu, Ce Bai Ye*<br>— Hemoptysis, subcutaneous and mucosa bleeding. *+ Bai Mao Gen, Xian He Cao* |
| **2. May be used in the treatment for hypertension.** |

[Dosage] 10-15 g. Often use the charred form.

[Comments] The alternative name is Huai Mi.

# Bai Mao Gen

*Rhizoma Imperatae*
*Sweet, cold; Lung, Stomach, Bladder*

[Characteristics] Cools the blood and stops bleeding. It is primarily used for hematuria. It also can clear heat, promote urination and generate fluid.

| FUNCTIONS • INDICATIONS & MAJOR COMBINATIONS |
| --- |
| **1. Cool the blood and stop bleeding:**<br>• Heat causing the blood to move recklessly with bleeding.<br>— Hematuria. *+ Ce Bai Ye*<br>— Bleeding at the upper part of the body. *+ Xian He Cao* |
| **2. Clear heat, promote urination and generate fluid:**<br>• Heat-type of Painful Urinary Dysfunction. *+ Che Qian Zi*<br>• Damp-heat jaundice. *+ Yin Chen Hao*<br>• Heat patterns with irritability and thirst or Stomach heat with vomiting. *+ Lu Gen* |

[Dosage] 10-15 g. May increase dose to 30-60 g. when using fresh herb.

# Qian Cao

*Radix Rubiae*
*Bitter, cold; Liver*

[Characteristics] Bitter and cold to clear heat, cool the blood and stop bleeding, it also transforms blood stasis to stop bleeding (fried form). It is primarily used for hemorrhaging due to heat causing reckless movement of the blood, as well as alleviating pain due to blood stasis.

**FUNCTIONS • INDICATIONS & MAJOR COMBINATIONS**

**1. Cool the blood and stop bleeding:**
- Widely used in various bleeding disorders due to heat causing the blood to move recklessly and traumatic injuries.

**2. Invigorate the blood and alleviate pain:**
- Blood stasis with amenorrhea. *+ Xiang Fu, Dang Gui*
- Traumatic injuries with swelling and pain. *+ Chuan Xiong, Hong Hua*
- Painful obstruction with joint pain. *+ Ji Xue Teng, Hai Feng Teng*

[Dosage] 10-15 g.

# Ce Bai Ye

*Cacumen Platycladi*
*Bitter, astringent, slightly cold; Lung, Liver, Large Intestine*

[Characteristics] It cools the blood to stop bleeding. Moreover, Ce Bai Ye is astringent in nature. It can clear the Lung, transform phlegm and stop coughing.

**FUNCTIONS • INDICATIONS & MAJOR COMBINATIONS**

**1. Cool the blood and stop bleeding:**
- Heat causing the blood to move recklessly with bleeding. *+ Da Ji, Bai Mao Gen*
- Deficient cold with bleeding. *+ Ai Ye, Pao Jiang*

**2. Expel phlegm and stop coughing:**
- Lung heat with cough and blood tinged sputum. *+ Huang Qin*

**3. For alopecia or small burn lesions, apply the herb topically.**

[Dosage] 10-15 g.

# Bai Ji

*Rhizoma Bletillae*
*Bitter, sweet, astringent, slightly cold; Lung, Stomach, Liver*

[Characteristics] With adhesive nature and astringent property, it is a powerful astringent hemostatic. It primarily treats hemorrhaging from the Lung and Stomach with hemoptysis and hematemesis, as well as trauma with bleeding. Bai Ji can be taken orally or applied topically. It also can promote healing and generate tissue for sores and carbuncles.

| FUNCTIONS • INDICATIONS & MAJOR COMBINATIONS |
|---|

**1. Astringe to stop bleeding:**
- Use this herb alone in powdered form could treat various types of hemorrhaging.
- Gastric bleeding with hematemesis or blood in the stool.
  *+ Hai Piao Xiao*
- Pulmonary bleeding with hemoptysis. *+ Pi Pa Ye, Ou Jie*
- Traumatic injuries with bleeding, topically apply the powdered mixture *+ Duan Shi Gao*

**2. Reduce swelling and generate tissue:**
- Sores and abscesses with or without perforation.
  — Early stage of or imperforated sores and abscesses. *+ Jin Yin Hua, Tian Hua Fen*
  — Perforated and non-healing sores and abscesses, topically apply the powdered form.
- Lung abscess with decreasing productive cough of foul smell and purulent bloody sputum. *+ Jin Yin Hua, Jie Geng*
- For burn lesions, cracked hand and feet with bleeding, apply the mixture of powdered Bai Ji and oil topically.

[Dosage] 3-10 g. 1.5-3 g. when using powdered form.

[Precautions] Incompatible with Wu Tou.

Herbs that Astringe to Stop Bleeding

# Xian He Cao

*Herba Agrimoniae*
*Bitter, astringent, neutral; Lung, Liver, Spleen*

[Characteristics] It is an astringent hemostatic herb. Being neutral in nature, it can be used in either cold or heat type of hemorrhaging. Xian He Cao can also astringe the intestines to stop diarrhea and kill parasites to stop itchiness.

**FUNCTIONS • INDICATIONS & MAJOR COMBINATIONS**

**1. Astringe to stop bleeding:**
- Widely used in various types of bleeding.
  — Heat in the blood. *+ Sheng Di Huang, Ce Bai Ye*
  — Deficient cold. *+ Huang Qi, Pao Jiang*

**2. Alleviate dysentery disorder and diarrhea:**
- Chronic diarrhea or dysentery disorder with blood in the stool.
  *+ Di Yu Tan, Huang Qin Tan*

**3. For external genital itchiness and increased discharge due to trichomoniasis vaginitis, use the concentrated decoction of Xian He Cao as a vaginal douche.**

[Dosage] 10-15 g. May increase the dose to 30-60 g.

# Ou Jie

*Nodus Nelumbinis Rhizomatis*
*Sweet, astringent, neutral; Lung, Liver, Stomach*

[Characteristics] It is astringent to stop bleeding; it also expels blood stasis. Ou Jie can stop bleeding without causing blood stasis. However, because of its relatively mild effects, it is mainly used as an auxiliary herb in prescriptions to treat various types of hemorrhaging.

**FUNCTIONS • INDICATIONS & MAJOR COMBINATIONS**

**Astringe to stop bleeding:**
- Widely used in various types of bleeding, especially effective in hematemesis and hemoptysis. *+ Bai Ji, Ce Bai Ye*

[Dosage] 10-15 g. Use raw form for invigorating the blood and stopping bleeding; charred form is astringent to stop bleeding.

# Pu Huang

*Pollen Typhae*
*Sweet, neutral; Heart, Liver*

[Characteristics] The raw form invigorates the blood to stop bleeding without causing blood stasis; charred form is astringent to stop bleeding. Pu Huang can be used in combination with other herbs for most types of hemorrhaging, regardless if the patterns are of cold or heat, deficiency or excess.

| FUNCTIONS • INDICATIONS & MAJOR COMBINATIONS |
| --- |
| **1. Stop bleeding:**<br>• Widely used in various types of bleeding. The charred form astringes to stop bleeding; the raw form invigorates the blood to stop bleeding. |
| **2. Invigorate the blood and alleviate pain:**<br>• Cardiac, chest and abdominal pain, post-partum abdominal pain and dysmenorrhea. *+ Wu Ling Zhi* |
| **3. Blood-type of Painful Urinary Dysfunction with hematuria.** |

[Dosage] 3-10 g. Seal in tea bags for decoction.

[Precautions] Contraindicated during pregnancy.


# San Qi

*Radix Notoginseng*
*Sweet, slightly bitter, warm; Liver, Stomach*

[Characteristics] San Qi is the imperial hemostatic that can be used for most types of bleeding. For conditions with blood stasis, it is especially effective. It also reduces swelling and alleviates pain. It is recognized as the imperial herb for traumatic injuries with hematoma, swelling and pain.

| FUNCTIONS • INDICATIONS & MAJOR COMBINATIONS |
| --- |
| **1. Transform blood stasis and stop bleeding:**<br>• Widely used in various types of bleeding, take the powdered form orally or apply it topically for bleeding due to traumatic injuries. |
| **2. Invigorate the blood and alleviate pain:**<br>• Traumatic injuries, chest pain or any pain related to blood stasis. |

[Dosage] 3-10 g. May reduce the dose to 1-1.5 g. when using powdered form.

# Ai Ye

*Folium Artemisiae Argyi*
*Bitter, acrid, warm; Liver, Spleen, Kidney*

[Characteristics] An acrid and warm herb, Ai Ye warms the meridians to stop bleeding as well as disperses cold to alleviate pain. It is often used for bleeding due to deficient cold, especially for gynecological disorders, such as Gushing and Leaking Syndromes, dysmenorrhea and irregular menstruation. Ai Ye is the primary herb for gynecological disorders. It is also a common herb for deficient cold with abdominal pain or wind-damp painful obstruction.

### FUNCTIONS • INDICATIONS & MAJOR COMBINATIONS

**1. Warm the meridians and stop bleeding:**
- Deficient cold with Gushing and Leaking Syndromes. Use the charred form or *+ E Jiao, Di Huang*
- Threatened miscarriage with spotting and Restless Fetus Syndromes. *+ Xu Duan, Sang Ji Sheng*

**2. Disperse cold and alleviate pain:**
- Lower burner deficient cold with abdominal cold pain and irregular menstruation. *+ Dang Gui, Xiang Fu*
- Middle burner deficient cold with cold pain in the epigastrium and abdomen. *+ Gan Jiang, Yan Hu Suo*

**3. For eczema and skin itchiness, use the decoction as an external wash.**

[Dosage] 3-10 g.

[Comments] The back of Ai Ye contains thick layers of fine hair, known as Ai Rong, or moxa wool, which is the material used to make moxa sticks or moxa cones. Clinically, moxa cones or moxa sticks are burned for moxibustion treatment. The funcitons of moxibustion include:

1) Warm the meridians to expel cold for cold types of painful obstruction.

2) Facilitate the smooth flow of qi and blood to lift yang qi.

3) Assist the yang to rescue collapsed qi and devastated yang.

4) Has prophylactic effects to promote health.

# Zao Xin Tu

*Terra Flava Usta*
*Acrid, warm; Spleen, Stomach*

[**Characteristics**] Mainly entering the middle burner, or the Spleen and Stomach, it warms the middle to stop bleeding, and is widely used for hemorrhaging due to Spleen deficient cold unable to hold the blood. It can also warm the middle to stop vomiting and diarrhea.

| FUNCTIONS • INDICATIONS & MAJOR COMBINATIONS |
| --- |
| **1. Warm the middle and stop bleeding:**<br>• Spleen deficient cold with sallow complexion, cold extremities, and hemorrhaging, such as hematemesis and blood in the stool, in which blood is dark in color. *+ Fu Zi, Di Huang* |
| **2. Warm the middle and stop vomiting:**<br>• Spleen and Stomach deficient cold with vomiting. *+ Ban Xia, Gan Jiang*<br>• Morning sickness with vomiting. *+ Zi Su Geng, Sha Ren* |
| **3. Warm the middle and stop diarrhea:**<br>• Spleen deficiency with chronic diarrhea. *+ Gan Jiang, Bai Zhu* |

[**Dosage**] 10-30 g. Seal in tea bags and decoct it first; may increase the dose to 60-120 g., and use the strained decoction to decoct other herbs in the prescription.

[**Comments**] The alternative name is Fu Long Gan.

## [Remarks & Differentiations]

### Di Yu — Huai Hua — Bai Mao Gen

|  | Di Yu | Huai Hua | Bai Mao Gen |
| --- | --- | --- | --- |
| **C** | Cool the blood and stop bleeding. | | |
| **D** | • Often combined for mutual reinforcement for blood in the stool and bleeding hemorrhoids. | | • Effectively treats hematuria.<br>• clears heat and promotes urination. |
| | • For burn lesions. | | |

# HERBS THAT
## Invigorate the Blood and Transform Stasis    11

Herbs in this chapter mainly unblock obstructions in the vessels, promote the circulation of blood, resolve and dispel stasis. In general, they are known as herbs that invigorate the blood and transform stasis. Some herbs are very powerful in breaking up blood stasis; they are known as herbs that break up stasis.

Its acrid and dispersing qualities help unblock obstructions in the blood vessels. These herbs facilitate the circulation of blood, regulate menstruation, dispel stasis to alleviate pain, reduce swelling, generate the tissue, and break up stasis to resolve *Zheng Jia Ji Ju*. They are used to treat patterns of internal and external pain caused by poor circulation and/or blood stasis, dysmenorrhea and amenorrhea due to blood stasis, hematoma and swelling due to traumatic injuries, and those of *Zheng Jia Ji Ju* and Wind-dampness Painful Obstruction.

Consider the phrases, "Qi is the commander of the blood" and "the circulation of blood follows the movement of qi" in the treatment principle. When using these herbs, it is recommended to combine other herbs that regulate the qi to enhance the therapeutic effects.

Herbs in this section should be used with caution, and are contraindicated for use in heavy menstrual flow and during pregnancy.

# Chuan Xiong

*Rhizoma Chuanxiong*
*Acrid, warm; Liver, Gallbladder, Pericardium*

[Characteristics] Acrid to disperse and warm to unblock, this herb enters both the blood and qi levels. Chuan Xiong is recognized as the "Qi herb in the blood level" because its primary functions are to invigorate the blood and promote the movement of qi. Moreover, ascending and dispersing in nature, it also dispels wind and alleviates pain; therefore, Chuan Xiong is the imperial herb for headache.

## FUNCTIONS • INDICATIONS & MAJOR COMBINATIONS

### 1. Invigorate the blood and promote the movement of qi:
- Patterns of qi stagnation and blood stasis. *+ Dang Gui*
- Blood stasis with irregular menstruation. *+ Xiang Fu, Chong Wei Zi*
- Liver qi stagnation and blood stasis with hypochondriac pain. *+ Chai Hu, Xiang Fu*
- Post-partum abdominal pain due to stasis. *+ Yi Mu Cao, Tao Ren*
- Traumatic injuries with blood stasis and pain. *+ Hong Hua, Ru Xiang*
- Deficient patterns of non-perforated sores, ulcers and toxic swelling. *+ Huang Qi, Jin Yin Hua*

### 2. Expel wind and alleviate pain:
- All patterns of headaches.
  — Exterior wind-cold. *+ Bai Zhi, Fang Feng*
  — Exterior wind-heat. *+ Ju Hua*
  — Exterior wind-dampness. *+ Qiang Huo, Fang Feng*
  — Blood stasis. *+ Chi Shao, Dan Shen*
- Wind-cold-damp Painful Obstruction. *+ Qiang Huo, Du Huo*

### 3. Commonly used as an herbal supplement in conditions of coronary arterial disease, angina, and/or ischemic cerebrovascular disease.

[Dosage] 3-10 g.

[Precautions] Not recommended for use in yin deficiency with heat or excessive menstruation and hemorrhaging.

[Comments] A classic blood invigorator, Chuan Xiong is widely used for various conditions of blood stasis. It possesses two functional tendencies. First, it is acrid and warm to ascend upward to act on the head for headaches, as in the ancient proverb, "to treat headache, Chuan Xiong has to be added." Second, it is also acrid and warm to unblock the obstruction, invigorate the blood, and reach downward to the origin of the Penetrating and Conception vessels for irregular menstruation.

# Dan Shen

*Radix Salviae Miltiorrhizae*
*Bitter, slightly cold; Heart, Pericardium, Liver*

[Characteristics] Dan Shen can be used for all patterns of blood stasis; however, slightly cold in nature, this herb can invigorate and cool the blood and is widely used to treat conditions of stasis with heat. Entering the Heart channel, Dan Shen clears heat from the Heart and nourishes the blood; it is commonly used in heat patterns of irritability and insomnia. Therefore, it is also recognized as an herb that can nourish the blood and calm the spirit.

| FUNCTIONS • INDICATIONS & MAJOR COMBINATIONS |
| --- |
| **1. Invigorate the blood and transform blood stasis:** <br> • Blood stasis with irregular menstruation and amenorrhea. <br>   *+ Chuan Xiong, Dang Gui* <br> • Blood stasis and qi stagnation with pain in the cardiac, chest, epigastric and abdominal regions. *+ Tan Xiang, Sha Ren* <br> • Chest Painful Obstruction due to blood stasis. *+ Yan Hu Suo, Chuan Xiong* <br> • *Zheng Jia Ji Ju*, such as hepatosplenomegaly. *+ San Leng, E Zhu* <br> • Traumatic injuries with painful limbs. *+ Hong Hua, Chuan Xiong* |
| **2. Cool the blood and reduce swelling:** <br> • Painful sores, abscesses and swelling or breast abscess. *+ Jin Yin Hua, Lian Qiao* |
| **3. Nourish the blood and calm the spirit:** <br> • Heat entering the nutritive and blood levels of Warm-Febrile Disease with high fever, irritability, insomnia and delirium. *+ Xuan Shen, Sheng Di Huang* <br> • Yin and blood deficiency or Heart and Kidney not communicating with insomnia and dream-disturbed sleep. *+ Suan Zao Ren, Yuan Zhi* |

[Dosage] 6-15 g. Frying with wine enhances the effect of invigorating the blood.

[Precautions] Incompatible with Li Lu.

[Comments] ❶ Dan Shen has been used as an herbal supplement in coronary arterial disease, angina and hepatosplenomegaly with good effects by adopting its function of invigorating the blood.

❷ According to the ancient proverb, "The function of Dan Shen is similar to Si Wu"; Si Wu, or the Four Substance Decoction, is a basic formula for nourishing and invigorating the blood.

# Chi Shao

*Radix Paeoniae Rubra*
*Bitter, slightly cold; Liver*

**[Characteristics]** Bitter and cold in nature, Chi Shao mainly enters the Liver channel, or the blood level; it cools and invigorates the blood. By cooling the blood, it is used for reckless movement of the blood in Warm-Febrile Disease with hemorrhaging; by invigorating the blood, it is used for patterns of blood stasis.

## FUNCTIONS • INDICATIONS & MAJOR COMBINATIONS

### 1. Invigorate the blood and dispel blood stasis:
- Blood deficiency and blood stasis with irregular menstruation. *+ Dang Gui, Chuan Xiong*
- Traumatic injuries with blood stasis and pain. *+ Tao Ren, Ru Xiang*
- Blood stasis with headache. *+ Chuan Xiong*

### 2. Clear heat and cool the blood:
- Heat entering the blood level in Warm-Febrile Disease, causing the blood to move recklessly with hematemesis, subcutaneous and mucosa bleeding. *+ Xi Jiao, Sheng Di Huang*

### 3. Cool the blood and reduce abscesses:
- Heat toxicity with abscesses and swelling. *+ Jin Yin Hua*
- Liver fire with red swollen painful eyes. *+ Ju Hua, Xia Ku Cao*

**[Dosage]** 6-15 g.

**[Precautions]** Incompatible with Li Lu.

**[Comments]** ❶ Chi Shao is a blood invigorator that is cold in nature; it is commonly combined with herbs that clear heat and cool the blood, such as Xi Jiao and Sheng Di Huang, for hemorrhages due to heat causing reckless movement of the blood. Recognizing its characteristic of "cooling the blood without causing stasis, and invigorating without disturbing the blood", it is therefore categorized into the herbs that clear heat and cool the blood in traditional textbooks.

❷ Chi Shao and Bai Shao were recognized as Shao Yao. In ancient documentations and applications, there were no obvious distinctions between Chi Shao and Bai Shao. However, there is a significant distinction between their individual functions. For differentiation and application (p. 219).

# Tao Ren

*Semen Persicae*
*Bitter, neutral; Heart, Liver, Lung, Large Intestine*

[Characteristics] A powerful herb with the effect of breaking up blood stasis, Tao Ren is an important herb for invigorating the blood and transforming blood stasis. It contains rich oil; therefore, it can moisten the intestines and unblock the obstruction of bowel movements.

| FUNCTIONS • INDICATIONS & MAJOR COMBINATIONS |
|---|
| **1. Invigorate the blood and dispel blood stasis:** |
|    • Blood stasis with amenorrhea, dysmenorrhea and post-partum abdominal pain. *+ Hong Hua, Dang Gui* |
|    • Traumatic injuries with blood stasis and pain. *+ Dang Gui, Da Huang* |
|    • Lung abscess. *+ Lu Gen, Dong Gua Ren* |
|    • Intestinal abscess. *+ Da Huang, Mu Dan Pi* |
| **2. Moisten the intestines and unblock the obstruction of bowel movements:** |
|    • Blood deficiency and intestinal dryness with constipation. *+ Huo Ma Ren, Gua Lou Ren* |
| **3. For coughing and wheezing, used as an auxiliary herb.** |

[Dosage] 6-10 g. Crush the herb before placing it in for decoction.

[Precautions] Contraindicated during pregnancy.

# Hong Hua

*Flos Carthami*
*Acrid, warm; Heart, Liver*

[Characteristics] Invigorating the blood and dispelling blood stasis, it is commonly combined with Tao Ren. Hong Hua is primarily used for gynecologic patterns of blood stasis as it is an important herb for invigorating the blood, regulating menstruation and alleviating pain.

**FUNCTIONS • INDICATIONS & MAJOR COMBINATIONS**

**1. Invigorate the blood and regulate menstruation:**
   - Blood stasis with amenorrhea, dysmenorrhea and post-partum abdominal pain. *+ Tao Ren, Dang Gui*

**2. Dispel blood stasis and alleviate pain:**
   - Patterns of pain due to blood stasis.
     — Chest Painful Obstruction with stabbing pain. *+ Dan Shen, Chuan Xiong*
     — Traumatic injuries with blood stasis and pain. *+ Ru Xiang, Mo Yao*
     — Sores, ulcers, swelling and pain. *+ Tao Ren, Chi Shao*
     — *Zheng Jia Ji Ju. + San leng, E Zhu*
   - Dark purplish purpura due to heat toxicity. *+ Zi Cao, Dang Gui*

[Dosage] 3-10 g.
[Precautions] Contraindicated during pregnancy.

[Addendum]
## Xi Hong Hua
**Stigma Croci**
The alternative name is Zang Hong Hua. Sweet and cold, it enters the Heart and Liver channels. Similar to Hong Hua, it can also invigorate the blood and dispel blood stasis but with stronger effects; it also can cool the blood and relieve toxicity, especially useful in heat patterns with dark purplish purpura, and incomplete expression of rashes from measles or heat in the blood level of Warm-Febrile Disease. Because of its expensive cost, it is rarely used clinically. 1.5-3 g.

# E Zhu

*Rhizoma Curcumae*
*Acrid, bitter, warm; Liver, Spleen*

[Characteristics] Entering the blood level, E Zhu is extremely effective in dispersing and moving. It invigorates the blood and breaks up blood stasis and it is mainly used for severe cases of qi stagnation and blood stasis, conditions known as *Zheng Jia Ji Ju*. It also enters the qi level to promote the movement of qi and break up the accumulations.

| FUNCTIONS • INDICATIONS & MAJOR COMBINATIONS |
|---|
| **1. Break up and dispel blood stasis:** <br> • Qi stagnation and blood stasis with amenorrhea, abdominal pain or *Zheng Jia Ji Ju.* *+ San Leng* |
| **2. Promote the movement of qi and break up accumulations:** <br> • Food retention and qi stagnation with epigastric and abdominal distention and pain. *+ San Leng, Zhi Shi* |

[Dosage] 3-10 g. Often processed with vinegar.

[Precautions] Contraindicated during pregnancy and heavy menstrual flow.


# San Leng

*Rhizoma Sparganii*
*Acrid, bitter, neutral; Liver, Spleen*

[Characteristics] Has similar effects as E Zhu, yet San Leng is stronger in breaking up blood stasis. For clinical use, San Leng is commonly combined with E Zhu for severe cases of qi stagnation and blood stasis, or *Zheng Jia Ji Ju.*

| FUNCTIONS • INDICATIONS & MAJOR COMBINATIONS |
|---|
| **1. Break up and dispel blood stasis:** <br> • Qi stagnation and blood stasis with amenorrhea and abdominal pain or *Zheng Jia Ji Ju.* *+ E Zhu* |
| **2. Promote the movement of qi and break up accumulations:** <br> • Food retention and qi stagnation with epigastric and abdominal distention and pain. *+ E Zhu, Qing Pi* |

[Dosage] 3-10 g. Often processed with vinegar.

[Precautions] Contraindicated during pregnancy and heavy menstrual flow.

# Ru Xiang

*Resina Olibani*
*Acrid, bitter, warm; Heart, Liver, Spleen*

[Characteristics] Invigorates the blood, promotes the movement of qi and alleviates pain. Ru Xiang is used for patterns of pain related to blood stasis. It is effective in reducing swelling and generating the tissue; therefore, it is commonly used for traumatic injuries with blood stasis and pain, non-healing ulcers and sores.

**FUNCTIONS • INDICATIONS & MAJOR COMBINATIONS**

**1. Invigorate the blood and alleviate pain:**
- Pain associated with qi stagnation and blood stasis. *+ Chuan Xiong*
- Traumatic injuries with blood stasis and pain. *+ Hong Hua, Mo Yao*
- Wind-cold-damp Painful Obstruction. *+ Qiang Huo, Du Huo*

**2. Reduce swelling and generate the tissue:**
- Toxic swelling, sores and abscesses with tender masses. *+ Mo Yao, She Xiang*
- For non-healing sores and ulcers, apply the powdered form topically.

[Dosage] 3-10 g. In most cases, this herb is applied topically.

[Precautions] Contraindicated during pregnancy.

# Mo Yao

*Myrrha*
*Bitter, neutral; Heart, Liver, Spleen*

[Characteristics] Has similar effects as Ru Xiang, yet Ru Xiang generally acts on the qi level while Mo Yao usually acts on the blood level. These two herbs are commonly combined for mutual reinforcement.

**FUNCTIONS • INDICATIONS & MAJOR COMBINATIONS**

**1. Invigorate the blood and alleviate pain:**
- Pain associated with qi stagnation and blood stasis. *+ Chuan Xiong*
- Traumatic injuries with blood stasis and pain. *+ Hong Hua, Ru Xiang*

**2. Reduce swelling and generate the tissue:**
- For non-healing sores and ulcers, apply the powdered form topically.

[Dosage] 3-10 g. In most cases, this herb is applied topically.

[Precautions] Contraindicated during pregnancy.

# Yi Mu Cao

*Herba Leonuri*
*Acrid, bitter, slightly cold; Heart, Liver, Bladder*

[Characteristics] Yi Mu Cao is literally translated into "the herb that benefits the female". It is primarily used for gynecologic disorders related to blood stasis. It promotes urination and reduces swelling, and is slightly cold in nature.

| FUNCTIONS • INDICATIONS & MAJOR COMBINATIONS |
| --- |
| **1. Invigorate the blood and expel stasis:**<br>• Gynecologic disorders related to blood stasis. Use the syrup form of this herb alone, or *+ Dang Gui, Chuan Xiong*<br>• Traumatic injuries with blood stasis and pain. *+ Dang Gui, Chi Shao* |
| **2. Promote urination and reduce swelling:**<br>• Dysuria and edema. *+ Bai Mao Gen* |

[Dosage] 10-30 g.

[Addendum]
## Chong Wei Zi
*Fructus Leonuri*
Sweet and slightly cold in nature, it has similar effects as Yi Mu Cao to invigorate the blood and regulate menstruation. It can also cool the Liver and brighten the eyes for Liver heat with red swollen painful eyes. 6-10 g.

# Ze Lan

*Herba Lycopi*
*Bitter, acrid, slightly warm; Liver, Spleen*

[Characteristics] Ze Lan invigorates the blood, expels stasis as well as promotes urination; has similar yet milder effects than Yi Mu Cao. It is warm in nature.

| FUNCTIONS • INDICATIONS & MAJOR COMBINATIONS |
| --- |
| **1. Invigorate the blood and expel blood stasis:**<br>• Gynecologic disorders related to blood stasis and traumatic injuries with blood stasis and pain. *+ Dang Gui, Chuan Xiong* |
| **2. Promote urination and reduce swelling for dysuria and edema.** |

[Dosage] 10-15 g.

# Yan Hu Suo

*Rhizoma Corydalis*
*Acrid, bitter, warm; Heart, Liver, Spleen*

[Characteristics] Invigorates the blood, promotes the movement of qi and alleviates pain. Yan Hu Suo is recognized as the Chinese herbal analgesic. It is used for all types of pain related to qi stagnation and blood stasis of any location.

**FUNCTIONS • INDICATIONS & MAJOR COMBINATIONS**

### Invigorate the blood, promote the movement of qi and alleviate pain:
- Pain associated with qi stagnation and blood stasis.
  — Epigastric and abdominal pain. *+ Chuan Lian Zi*
  — Dysmenorrhea. *+ Chuan Xiong, Dang Gui*
  — Chest Painful Obstruction with stabbing pain. *+ Dan Shen*
  — Hernia disorder with pain. *+ Wu Yao, Xiao Hui Xiang*
  — Traumatic injuries. *+ Ru Xiang, Mo Yao*

[Dosage] 6-10 g. Reduce to 1.5-3 g when using the powdered form. To process with vinegar enhances its analgesic effect.

[Comments] ❶ The alternative name is Yuan Hu.

❷ Yan Hu Suo is often combined with Dan Shen and Chuan Xiong to help treat coronary arterial disease and alleviate angina with good result.

# Wu Ling Zhi

*Excrementum Trogopteri seu Pteromi*
*Bitter, sweet, warm; Liver*

[Characteristics] An important herb for invigorating the blood and alleviating pain, it is used for patterns of pain due to blood stasis.

**FUNCTIONS • INDICATIONS & MAJOR COMBINATIONS**

### 1. Invigorate the blood and alleviate pain:
- Blood stasis with pain. *+ Pu Huang*

### 2. Transform blood stasis and stop bleeding:
- Blood stasis with bleeding. *+ San Qi*

[Dosage] 6-10 g. Seal in tea bags for decoction. Raw form invigorates blood; fried form stops bleeding.

[Precautions] Antagonized with Ren Shen. Contraindicated during pregnancy.

# Yu Jin

*Radix Curcumae*
*Acrid, bitter, cold; Heart, Liver, Gallbladder*

**[Characteristics]** Acrid to move, bitter to drain, and cold to clear heat, Yu Jin enters the Liver channel to invigorate the blood and promote the movement of qi for blood stasis and qi stagnation with chest, hypochondriac and abdominal pain. It enters the Heart channel to cool the blood and clear the Heart for heat patterns with loss of consciousness. Yu Jin also enters the Liver and Gallbladder to drain dampness and reduce jaundice for damp-heat jaundice.

| FUNCTIONS • INDICATIONS & MAJOR COMBINATIONS |
| --- |
| **1. Invigorate the blood and promote the movement of qi:**<br>• Constrained Liver qi and blood stasis with hypochondriac distention and pain. *+ Chai Hu, Xiang Fu*<br>• Hypochondriac *Zheng Jia* due to qi stagnation and blood stasis. *+ Bie Jia, Qing Pi* |
| **2. Cool the blood and clear the Heart:**<br>• Damp-warm Febrile Disease when turbid phlegm obstructs the Heart's orifice manifesting with disorientation or mental derangement. *+ Shi Chang Pu*<br>• Heat entering the nutritive and blood levels in Warm-Febrile Disease with irritability, delirium and unconsciousness. *+ Huang Lian* |
| **3. Benefit the gallbladder and reduce jaundice:**<br>• Damp-heat jaundice. *+ Yin Chen Hao, Zhi Zi* |
| **4. Used in heat causing the blood to move recklessly with hemoptysis, hematemesis, subcutaneous and mucosa bleeding.** |

**[Dosage]** 6-10 g.

**[Precautions]** Antagonized with Ding Xiang.

# Niu Xi

*Radix Achyranthis Bidentatae seu Cyathulae*
*Bitter, sour, neutral; Liver, Kidney*

[Characteristics] Invigorating the blood to dispel stasis as well as directing the blood and heat downward, Niu Xi is primarily used for conditions of amenorrhea due to blood stasis, hematemesis or subcutaneous and mucosa bleeding due to heat in the blood, and for Heat-type and Blood-type of Painful Urinary Dysfunction. Moreover, it tonifies the Liver and Kidney to strengthen the sinews and bones; it treats soreness and weakness of the lower back and knees with good results.

**FUNCTIONS • INDICATIONS & MAJOR COMBINATIONS**

### 1. Invigorate the blood and dispel stasis:
- Blood stasis with dysmenorrhea, amenorrhea and irregular menstruation. *+ Tao Ren, Hong Hua*
- Traumatic injuries, blood stasis and pain at the lower back and knees. *+ Chuan Xiong, Xu Duan*

### 2. Tonify the Liver and Kidney to strengthen the lower back and knees:
- Soreness and weakness or pain at the lower back and knees.
  — Insufficiency of the Liver and Kidney. *+ Du Zhong, Sang Ji Sheng*
  — Deficiency and consumption disorder. *+ Shu Di Huang, Gui Ban*
  — Damp-heat infusing downward. *+ Cang Zhu, Huang Bai*
  — Wind-damp Painful Obstruction. *+ Mu Gua, Du Huo*

### 3. Guide the movement of blood downward:
- Heat causing the blood to move recklessly with bleeding of the upper body. *+ Bai Mao Gen, Zhi Zi*
- Yin deficiency with heat signs, such as toothache and sores in the mouth. *+ Shu Di Huang, Shi Gao*
- Liver yang rising with dizziness and tinnitus. *+ Mu Li, Long Gu*

### 4. Promote urination and unblock the obstruction in the urinary tract, used for Heat-type or Blood-type of Painful Urinary Dysfunction.

[Dosage] 6-15 g.

[Precautions] Contraindicated during pregnancy and excessive menstruation.

[Comments] There are two types of Niu Xi— Chuan Niu Xi, and Huai Niu Xi:

**Chuan Niu Xi** is effective to invigorate the blood and dispel stasis.

**Huai Niu Xi** is much stronger in tonifying the Liver and Kidney to strengthen the sinews and bones.

# Ji Xue Teng

*Caulis Spatholobi*
*Bitter, sweet, warm; Liver*

[Characteristics] Acrid to move the blood and sweet to nourish the blood, Ji Xue Teng is an herb that can invigorate and tonify the blood; it can also relax the sinews and unblock the collaterals. Therefore, it is especially appropriate for conditions of blood stasis and blood deficiency.

| FUNCTIONS • INDICATIONS & MAJOR COMBINATIONS |
| --- |
| **1. Invigorate and tonify the blood:**<br>• Irregular menstruation, dysmenorrhea and amenorrhea.<br>— Blood stasis. *+ Chuan Xiong, Hong Hua*<br>— Blood deficiency. *+ Shu Di Huang, Dang Gui* |
| **2. Relax the senews and unblock the collaterals:**<br>• Wind-dampness Painful Obstruction, or soreness and pain of the joints and numbness of the extremities. *+ Du Huo, Qin Jiao*<br>• Hemiplegia status post wind stroke. *+ Huang Qi, Di Long* |

[Dosage] 10-30 g.


# Jiang Huang

*Rhizoma Curcumae Longae*
*Acrid, bitter, warm; Liver, Spleen*

[Characteristics] Has similar effects as E Zhu, Jiang Huang invigorates the blood and promotes the movement of qi. It effectively acts on the upper extremities to invigorate the blood and dispel wind for Wind-dampness Painful Obstruction.

| FUNCTIONS • INDICATIONS & MAJOR COMBINATIONS |
| --- |
| **1. Break up blood stasis and promote the movement of qi:**<br>• Pain associated with qi stagnation and blood stasis. *+ Yan Hu Suo* |
| **2. For Wind-cold-damp Painful Obstruction, especially of the upper extremities and shoulders. It can invigorate the blood, dispel wind and alleviate pain.** *+ Qiang Huo, Hai Tong Pi* |
| **3. For toxic swelling, sores and carbuncles, apply topically.** |

[Dosage] 6-10 g.

# Wang Bu Liu Xing

*Semen Vaccariae*
*Bitter, neutral; Liver, Stomach*

[Characteristics] Acrid in nature, entering the blood level, this herb strongly moves without settling. Therefore, Wang Bu Liu Xing is an herb that invigorates the blood, regulates menstruation and promotes lactation.

**FUNCTIONS • INDICATIONS & MAJOR COMBINATIONS**

**1. Invigorate the blood and regulate menstruation:**
   • Blood stasis with dysmenorrhea and amenorrhea. *+ Chuan Xiong*

**2. Promote lactation:**
   • Insufficient lactation due to deficiency. *+ Huang Qi, Dang Gui*
   • Breast abscess with swelling and pain. *+ Xia Ku Cao, Gua Lou*

[Dosage] 6-10 g.

[Precautions] Contraindicated during pregnancy.

[Comments] ❶ The alternative name is Wang Bu Liu.

❷ Wang Bu Liu Xing has been used for auricular acupressure.

# Chuan Shan Jia

*Squama Manis*
*Salty, slightly cold; Liver, Stomach*

[Characteristics] Chuan Shan Jia specifically moves and disperses with strong effects of invigorating the blood and regulating menstruation. It can also promote lactation, reduce swelling and promote purulent discharge.

**FUNCTIONS • INDICATIONS & MAJOR COMBINATIONS**

**1. Invigorate the blood and regulate menstruation:**
   • Blood stasis with dysmenorrhea and amenorrhea. *+ Chuan Xiong*
   • Blood stasis with *Zheng Jia Ji Ju*. *+ San Leng, E Zhu*

**2. Promote lactation for insufficient lactation and breast abscess.**

**3. Reduce swelling and promote purulent discharge:**
   • Early stage or non-perforated suppurated abscesses. *+ Zao Jiao Ci*

[Dosage] 3-10 g. Powdered form is more effective; may reduce to 1-1.5 g.

[Precautions] Contraindicated during pregnancy.

# Xue Jie

*Sanguis Draxonis*
*Sweet, salty, neutral; Heart, Liver*

**[Characteristics]** Xue Jie is an important herb with a strong analgesic effect for pain due to traumatic injuries. It helps generate the tissue for skin ulcers and sores by invigorating the blood to promote healing. It has dual functions of stopping bleeding as well as promoting the circulation of blood for blood stasis.

| FUNCTIONS • INDICATIONS & MAJOR COMBINATIONS |
| --- |
| **1. Stop bleeding, generate the tissue and promote healing:**<br>• Traumatic injuries with bleeding. Apply the powdered form topically. *+ Pu Huang*<br>• Non-healing ulcers. *+ Ru Xiang, Mo Yao*<br>• Traumatic injuries with hematoma and pain. *+ Er Cha, Bing Pian* |
| **2. Invigorate the blood and alleviate pain:**<br>• Blood stasis with amenorrhea, dysmenorrhea and stabbing pain in the chest and abdomen. *+ Dang Gui, San Leng* |

**[Dosage]** 1-1.5 g. Add powder to pills.

## [Remarks & Differentiations]

**Tao Ren and Hong Hua /**
**E Zhu and San Leng /**
**Ru Xiang and Mo Yao:**
These three pairs of herbs are grouped together based on their shared functions and are usually combined to enhance their therapeutic effects. However, the herbs from each pair are different in strength to invigorate the blood and transform blood stasis.

**Yi Mu Cao and Ze Lan:**
Sharing the same effects, the difference lies on their individual temperature.

**Yan Hu Suo and Wu Ling Zhi:**
These two herbs are classic analgesic herbs that invigorate the blood and transform stasis.

**Dan Shen and Ji Xue Teng:**
They also nourish the blood while invigorate the blood; they are commonly used for blood stasis accompanied by blood deficiency.

**Chi Shao, Yu Jin, Dan Shen and Yi Mu Cao:**
These herbs are cold in nature; they cool the blood as well as invigorate the blood; therefore, they work well in blood stasis with heat signs.

**Ru Xiang, Mo Yao and Xue Jie:**
They can be taken orally or applied topically for blood stasis with swelling and pain due to traumatic injuries.

**Dan Shen and Yu Jin:**

Both invigorate the blood and transform stasis, cool the blood, clear pathogenic influences from the Heart and eliminate irritability. The former clears heat and nourishes the Heart to calm the spirit, while the latter clears turbid phlegm from the Heart's orifice to calm the spirit.

**E Zhu, San Leng and Chuan Shan Jia:**

Invigorating the blood and breaking up blood stasis, they are used for severe cases of *Zheng Jia Ji Ju.*

# HERBS THAT
## Warm the Interior 12

By warming and dispersing cold internally, herbs in this category treat patterns of interior cold. They are acrid and hot. Some herbs warm the middle burner, strengthen the Spleen and Stomach, dispel cold and alleviate pain; they are used to treat cold invading the interior and hindering the Spleen and Stomach yang qi with symptoms of cold pain in the epigastrium and abdomen, vomiting and diarrhea. Some herbs assist to rescue the devastated yang and reverse peripheral frigidity; they are used for exhausted yang qi and internal excessive cold with icy-cold extremities, minute or faint pulse, and for pattern of devastated yang and collapsed qi.

Herbs that warm the interior are commonly combined with herbs that warm and tonify the Spleen and Kidney. They are combined with herbs that strongly tonify the basal qi in conditions of devastated yang and collapsed qi.

Because of their acrid, hot and drying nature, these herbs should be used with caution. It is contraindicated for use in excess heat, yin deficiency and during pregnancy.

# Fu Zi

*Radix Aconiti Lateralis Preparata*
*Acrid, hot, toxic; Heart, Kidney, Spleen*

[Characteristics] Extremely acrid and hot, Fu Zi has the nature of pure yang to act on all twelve channels. It assists the Heart yang, warms the Spleen yang, tonifies the Kidney yang, disperses cold and alleviates pain. It is the imperial herb to tonify the fire and disperse cold, as well as restore devastated yang and reverse peripheral frigidity. It is used in all true cold patterns regardless of the location.

## FUNCTIONS • INDICATIONS & MAJOR COMBINATIONS

### 1. Restore devastated yang to reverse peripheral frigidity:
- Devastated yang with perspiration and clammy skin, icy-cold extremities and faint or minute pulse. *+ Gan Jiang, Zhi Gan Cao*
- Devastated yang and/or collapsed qi with extremely pale complexion, abundant perspiration and shortness of breath. *+ Ren Shen*

### 2. Tonify the fire and assist the yang:
- Patterns of yang deficiency.
  — Kidney yang insufficiency. *+ Rou Gui, Shu Di Huang*
  — Spleen yang insufficiency. *+ Ren Shen, Gan Jiang*
  — Deficient Spleen and Kidney yang with edema. *+ Bai Zhu*

### 3. Disperse cold, warm the channels and alleviate pain:
- Wind-cold-damp Painful Obstruction. *+ Gui Zhi, Bai Zhu*

[Dosage] 3-15 g. To minimize toxicity, decoct Fu Zi first for 30-60 minutes prior to adding in the other ingredients from the formula.

[Precautions] Contraindicated during pregnancy and incompatible with Ban Xia, Gua Lou, Tian Hua Fen, Bei Mu, Bai Ji and Bai Lian.

[Addendum]
## Wu Tou
*Radix Aconiti*

There are two types of Wu Tou— Chuan Wu and Cao Wu:

**Chuan Wu**, acrid, bitter, warm and very toxic, it enters the Heart, Liver and Spleen channels. Compared to Fu Zi, it has relatively stronger effects to dispel wind-dampness, disperse cold and alleviate pain. Process first before administrating. 3-10 g. Refer to Fu Zi for application methods and precautions.

**Cao Wu** has the same properties, effects, applications and precautions as Chuan Wu, but it is more toxic. 1.5-3 g.

# Rou Gui

*Cortex Cinnamomi*
*Acrid, sweet, hot; Heart, Kidney, Liver, Spleen*

[Characteristics] Acrid, extremely hot and sweet in nature, it is considered an herb with pure yang nature. Compared to Fu Zi, Rou Gui is slightly weaker in its ability to tonify the fire and disperse cold. It has relatively gentler but longer lasting effects. It is the imperial herb for leading the fire back to its source. It is often used in Spleen and Kidney yang deficiency, failure of fire in the Gate of Vitality, pain due to congealed cold and deficient yang floating upward.

| FUNCTIONS • INDICATIONS & MAJOR COMBINATIONS |
| --- |

**1. Tonify the fire, assist the yang and guide the fire back to its source:**
- Kidney yang deficiency, or the failure of fire in the Gate of Vitality. *+ Fu Zi, Shu Di Huang*
- Spleen and Kidney yang deficiency. *+ Fu Zi, Gan Jiang*
- Deficient yang floating upward due to lower burner deficient cold, or heat above and cold below.

**2. Disperse cold and alleviate pain:**
- Congealed cold causing qi stagnation with pain. *+ Xiao Hui Xiang, Wu Yao*
- Congealed cold causing blood stasis with pain or dysmenorrhea. *+ Chuan Xiong, Dang Gui*

**3. Warm and unblock the channels and vessels:**
- Yin-type of boils or non-healing sores. *+ Di Huang, Huang Qi*

**4. Use with herbs that tonify the qi and nourish the blood to promote the generation of the qi and blood.**

[Dosage] 3-6 g. Should not be decocted for long periods of time. 1-2 g. when using the powdered form.

[Precautions] Contraindicated in yin deficiency with heat signs, heat causing the blood to move recklessly with bleeding, and during pregnancy.

[Comments] Rou Gui is the bark and Gui Zhi is the branch of the plant, cinnamon. Both can warm the yang and disperse cold. Rou Gui disperses internal cold to alleviate pain; it mainly enters the lower burner to tonify Kidney yang. Gui Zhi releases the exterior and disperses cold; it mainly acts upward, facilitates the movement of qi and blood, warms the channels and unblocks the flow of yang.

# Gan Jiang

*Rhizoma Zingiberis*
*Acrid, hot; Spleen, Stomach, Heart, Lung*

**[Characteristics]** Extremely acrid, hot and drying, but non-toxic, it mainly enters the middle burner; therefore, Gan Jiang is the primary herb for warming the middle and expelling cold. It also warms the Lung and transforms congested fluids. Moreover, it is used as an auxiliary herb to restore devastated yang.

### FUNCTIONS • INDICATIONS & MAJOR COMBINATIONS

**1. Warm the middle and expel cold:**
- Deficient cold of the middle burner with cold pain in the epigastrium and abdomen, lack of appetite and loose stool. *+ Dang Shen, Bai Zhu*
- Excess cold of the middle burner with epigastric and abdominal pain, nausea and vomiting. *+ Gao Liang Jiang*

**2. Warm the Lung and transform congested fluids:**
- Cold congested fluids hidden in the Lung with wheezing and coughing up copious watery sputum. *+ Xi Xin, Wu Wei Zi*

**3. Restore devastated yang:**
- Devastated yang with icy-cold extremities, perspiration, clammy skin, and faint or minute pulse. *+ Fu Zi, Zhi Gan Cao*

**[Dosage]** 3-10 g.

**[Precautions]** Use with caution during pregnancy.

**[Comments]** Gan Jiang is the dried form of ginger and Sheng Jiang is the fresh form. They have different properties and effects. Sheng Jiang is acrid and warm; releasing the exterior, warming the middle and stopping vomiting, it treats exterior wind-cold and vomiting due to Stomach cold. Gan Jiang is acrid and hot, and it has strong effects to warm the middle, disperse cold, as well as warm the Lung and transform congested fluids; it is often used for deficient cold in the middle burner, wheezing and coughing due to cold congested fluids hidden in the Lung.

## [Addendum]
## Pao Jiang
### *Rhizoma Zingiberis Preparatum*
The fried form of ginger that is slightly scorched at the surface, bitter, astringent and warm, it enters the Liver and Spleen channels. It has similar effects as Gan Jiang. Less effective in warming the interior, it warms the channels to stop bleeding with good results. It is often used for bleeding due to deficient cold. 3-6 g.

# Wu Zhu Yu

*Fructus Evodiae*
*Acrid, bitter, hot, slightly toxic; Liver, Spleen, Stomach*

**[Characteristics]** Acrid to disperse and spread Liver qi, bitter to descend and direct rebellious qi down, hot to warm and assist the yang, Wu Zhu Yu warms Spleen and Stomach of the middle burner, as well as Liver and Kidney of the lower burner to alleviate pain and stop vomiting. It is the imperial herb for patterns of cold lodged in the Liver channel.

**FUNCTIONS • INDICATIONS & MAJOR COMBINATIONS**

**1. Disperse cold and alleviate pain:**
- Cold lodged in the Liver channel with vertex headache, dry heaves or vomiting up clear fluids. *+ Ren Shen, Sheng Jiang*
- Cold lodged in the Liver channel with hernia pain along the Liver channel. *+ Wu Yao, Xiao Hui Xiang*
- Deficient cold of the Penetrating and Conception vessels with irregular menstruation accompanied with cold pain in the lower abdomen. *+ Gui Zhi, Chuan Xiong*
- Yang deficiency of the Spleen and Kidney with daybreak diarrhea. *+ Bu Gu Zhi, Rou Dou Kou*

**2. Soothe the Liver and redirect rebellious qi downward:**
- Liver fire invading the Stomach with distention and pain in the epigastric and hypochondriac regions, vomiting, acid regurgitation and bitter taste in the mouth. *+ Huang Lian*

**[Dosage]** 1.5-6 g. It is not for chronic use. When made into powder form and mixed with vinegar, it can be topically applied on the soles of the feet to lead the fire downward and treat sores of the mouth and tongue.

**[Precautions]** Contraindicated in yin deficiency with heat signs.

**[Comments]** Wu Zhu Yu is an extremely hot herb, but still could be used in heat pattern of Liver fire invading the Stomach when it is combined with Huang Lian, which is bitter and cold in nature to clear heat and drain fire. This combination takes advantage of Wu Zhu Yu's effects to soothe constrained Liver qi and redirect rebellious qi down. Its hot nature moderates the cold nature of Huang Lian; moreover, it is also a guiding herb.

# Gao Liang Jiang

*Rhizoma Alpiniae Officinarum*
*Acrid, hot; Spleen, Stomach*

**[Characteristics]** Mainly entering the Spleen and Stomach, Gao Liang Jiang primarily disperses excess cold from the middle burner; it can also alleviate pain, descend rebellious qi and stop vomiting. It is often used for pain or vomiting due to cold congealing and qi stagnation.

**FUNCTIONS • INDICATIONS & MAJOR COMBINATIONS**

**Warm the middle, disperse cold and alleviate pain:**
- Cold congealing and qi stagnation with epigastric and abdominal pain. *+ Xiang Fu*
- Epigastric and abdominal cold pain with diarrhea. *+ Gan Jiang*
- Stomach cold with nausea and vomiting. *+ Sheng Jiang, Ban Xia*

**[Dosage]** 3-10 g.

**[Comments]** Both Gao Liang Jiang and Sheng Jiang warm the middle and disperse cold. Sheng Jiang is categorized into acrid and warm herbs that release the exterior; it primarily releases the exterior; it can also warm the middle and stop vomiting. In comparison, Gao Liang Jiang is acrid and hot, and tends to act on the interior; it primarily disperses Stomach cold and alleviates pain.


# Hua Jiao

*Pericarpium Zanthoxyli*
*Acrid, hot, slightly toxic; Spleen, Stomach, Kidney*

**[Characteristics]** Warms the middle and disperses cold to alleviate pain, as well as warms the Spleen to stop diarrhea. It can also eradicate the parasites.

**FUNCTIONS • INDICATIONS & MAJOR COMBINATIONS**

**1. Warm the middle and disperse cold:**
- Deficient cold of the Spleen and Stomach with cold pain in the epigastrium and abdomen, and vomiting. *+ Ren Shen, Gan Jiang*
- Cold-damp diarrhea. *+ Cang Zhu, Hou Po*

**2. Abdominal pain due to roundworms.**

**[Dosage]** 3-6 g.

**[Comments]** The alternative name is Chuan Jiao.

# Xiao Hui Xiang

*Fructus Foeniculi*
*Acrid, warm; Liver, Kidney, Spleen, Stomach*

[**Characteristics**] It disperses cold as well as facilitates the movement of qi. It acts on the middle and lower burner; it is the imperial herb for cold hernia disorder.

| FUNCTIONS • INDICATIONS & MAJOR COMBINATIONS |
| --- |
| **1. Disperse cold and alleviate pain:** <br> • Hernia disorder with lower abdominal cold pain. Wrap the fried herb in a cloth and use it as a warm compression or *+ Wu Yao* <br> • Liver qi stagnation with testicular distended pain. *+ Ju He, Shan Zha* |
| **2. Facilitate the movement of qi and harmonize the Stomach:** <br> • Stomach cold with vomiting and abdominal pain. *+ Gan Jiang* |

[**Dosage**] 3-6 g.

# Ding Xiang

*Flos Caryophylli*
*Acrid, warm; Spleen, Stomach, Kidney*

[**Characteristics**] Aromatic in nature, it enters the Spleen and Stomach, and warms the middle burner. Characterized by its ability to redirect Stomach qi downwards, it is an important herb for Stomach cold with nausea and vomiting. It can also warm the lower burner and assist the yang.

| FUNCTIONS • INDICATIONS & MAJOR COMBINATIONS |
| --- |
| **1. Warm the middle and direct rebellious qi downwards:** <br> • Deficient cold with hiccup and vomiting. *+ Ren Shen, Gan Jiang* <br> • Excess cold with hiccup and vomiting. *+ Ban Xia* |
| **2. Warm the Kidney and assist the yang:** <br> • Kidney yang deficiency with impotence. *+ Fu Zi, Rou Gui* |

[**Dosage**] 3-6 g.

[**Precautions**] Antagonized with Yu Jin.

[**Comments**] There are two types of Ding Xing in clinical applications:

> **Gong Ding Xiang** has rapid onset of action and stronger effects.
>
> **Mu Ding Xiang** has slow onset of action yet lasts longer.

## [Remarks & Differentiations]

### Fu Zi — Rou Gui

|   | **Fu Zi** | **Rou Gui** |
|---|---|---|
| **C** | Warm the interior and dispel cold. Tonify the fire and assist the yang. Combined for mutual reinforcement in interior cold. ||
| **D** | • Strong actions, the imperial herb for restoring devastated yang to reverse peripheral frigidity.<br>• Extremely acrid, drying and aggressive, moves without settling to strongly disperse cold, commonly used in critical conditions. | • Milder actions, the imperial herb for leading the floating fire back to its source.<br>• Acrid and sweet, it moves as well as settles, often combined with other tonics. |

### Fu Zi — Wu Tou

|   | **Fu Zi** | **Wu Tou** |
|---|---|---|
| **C** | From the same plant; acrid, hot and toxic. Warm the interior and dispel cold. ||
| **D** | • Tonifies the fire and assists the yang, often used to restore devastated yang and reverse peripheral frigidity. | • Dispels wind-dampness, disperses cold and alleviates pain, often used for Wind-dampness Painful Obstruction. |

### Fu Zi — Gan Jiang

|   | **Fu Zi** | **Gan Jiang** |
|---|---|---|
| **C** | Acrid and hot to warm the interior and disperse cold. Combined for mutual reinforcement to restore devastated yang and reverse peripheral frigidity. ||
| **D** | • Mainly enters the Kidney channel to tonify the fire and assist the yang.<br><br>• Disperses wind-dampness and alleviates pain. | • Mainly enters the middle burner, or the Spleen and Stomach, to warm the middle and disperse cold.<br>• Warms the Lung and transforms congested fluids. |

## Gan Jiang — Gao Liang Jiang

|   | Gan Jiang | Gao Liang Jiang |
|---|-----------|-----------------|
| C | Acrid and hot to warm the middle and disperse cold. | |
| D | • Warms the Spleen to treat Spleen deficient cold with abdominal pain and diarrhea. | • Warms the Stomach and disperses cold to treat Stomach cold with abdominal pain and vomiting. |

## Wu Zhu Yu — Gan Jiang

|   | Wu Zhu Yu | Gan Jiang |
|---|-----------|-----------|
| C | Enter the Spleen and Stomach to warm the middle and disperse cold. | |
| D | • Enters the Liver at the lower burner to disperse cold and alleviate pain for cold-type of hernia disorder. | • Enters the Lung at the upper burner to warm the Lung and transform congested fluids. |

## Xiao Hui Xiang — Ding Xiang

|   | Xiao Hui Xiang | Ding Xiang |
|---|----------------|------------|
| C | Disperse cold and facilitate the movement of qi. Warm the middle to redirect rebellious qi and stop vomiting. | |
| D | • Mainly enters the Liver channel to disperse cold for cold-type of hernia disorder. | • Also enters the Kidney channel to warm the Kidney and assist yang for impotence. |

# HERBS THAT
## Calm the Spirit                    13

These herbs primarily calm the spirit. They can be further subcategorized into two groups: (1) herbs that anchor, settle and calm the spirit and (2) herbs that nourish the Heart and calm the spirit. The former consists of mainly mineral substances. Its cold nature and heavy quality helps clear fire and subdue floating yang. They are used to treat Heart fire blazing up or Liver yang disturbing up with restlessness, irritability and insomnia. Herbs that nourish the Heart and calm the spirit consists of mainly seeds. They contain rich oil and are moist in nature to nourish the Heart and calm the spirit. This group of herbs can be used to treat qi and blood deficiency, or malnourishment of the mind, with palpitation, insomnia and forgetfulness.

Herbs that clear and drain fire from the Heart, pacify the Liver and subdue the yang or herbs that tonify the qi and blood are usually combined with herbs from this category to increase the tranquilizing effect.

Mineral substances have adverse effects on the Spleen and Stomach and they are not recommended for long-term use; they should be taken with herbs that strengthen the middle burner. Some herbs from this group also contain heavy metal; they are toxic and should be used with extreme caution.

# Zhu Sha

*Cinnabaris*
*Sweet, cold; Heart*

[Characteristics] A sweet, cold and heavy mineral, Zhu Sha mainly enters the Heart channel. The cold characteristic drains fire while the heaviness sedates the Heart; therefore, it is the imperial herb for clearing Heart fire and soothing the mind. In the patterns of disturbed spirit due to excessive Heart fire, this herb is usually added. When it is used as a processing material, it can enhance the effects of other tranquilizing herbs. Also, it has additional effects of clearing heat and relieving toxicity when taken orally or applied topically.

| FUNCTIONS • INDICATIONS & MAJOR COMBINATIONS |
|---|
| **1. Sedate the Heart and calm the spirit:** |
| • Heart fire blazing and disturbing the spirit with restlessness, agitation, irritability, hot sensation in the chest, panic with palpitation, anxiety and insomnia. *+ Huang Lian, Sheng Di Huang* |
| • High fever, delirium and loss of consciousness. *+ Xi Jiao, Niu Huang* |
| • Blood deficiency with palpitation and insomnia. *+ Bai Zi Ren, Suan Zao Ren* |
| • Seizures. *+ Ci Shi, Shen Qu* |
| **2. Clear heat and relieve toxicity:** |
| • Heat toxicity with swollen sore throat, sores in the mouth and tongue. *+ Bing Pian, Peng Sha* |
| • Heat toxicity with sores and carbuncles. *+ Xiong Huang* |
| **3. Used as a preservative to coat the pills.** |

[Dosage] 0.3-1 g. Add the powdered form into the strained decoction or make into pill form.

[Precautions] To prevent mercury poisoning, this herb is not to exceed the recommended dose or to be used long-term. Contraindicated in patients with liver and kidney abnormalities. Do not calcine.

[Comments] ❶ The alternative name is Chen Sha.

❷ To treat insomnia due to Heart fire excess, Zhu Sha is often combined with Huang Lian. Zhu Sha, sweet, cold and heavy in nature, strongly sedates and calms the spirit; Huang Lian, bitter and cold in nature, powerfully drains fire. Combined together for mutual assistance, their therapeutic effects are enhanced.

# Ci Shi

*Magnetitum*
*Acrid, salty, cold; Heart, Liver, Kidney*

[Characteristics] Salty, cold and heavy, it descends downward. Entering the Heart channel, Ci Shi drains Heart fire and soothes the mind; entering the Liver channel, it nourishes Liver yin and subdues Liver yang; entering the Kidney channel, it assists the Kidney to grasp the qi and improves visual and auditory acuities. Ci Shi is commonly used for heat disturbing upward with irritability and insomnia or Liver and Kidney yin deficiency with dull vision, tinnitus and deficient wheezing.

| FUNCTIONS • INDICATIONS & MAJOR COMBINATIONS |
| --- |
| **1. Anchor floating yang and calm the spirit:**<br>• Yin deficiency and yang rising with palpitation, insomnia and irritability. *+ Zhu Sha*<br>• Yin deficiency and yang rising with dizziness, vertigo and headaches. *+ Long Gu, Mu Li* |
| **2. Improve visual and auditory acuities:**<br>• Liver and Kidney yin deficiency with dull vision, tinnitus, impaired hearing or deafness. *+ Shu Di Huang, Shan Zhu Yu* |
| **3. Assist the Kidney to grasp the qi and calm wheezing:**<br>• Kidney deficiency unable to grasp the qi with deficient wheezing. *+ Wu Wei Zi, Hu Tao Rou* |

[Dosage] 10-30 g. Crush and decoct first, or add the powder into pills.

[Precautions] Not recommended to take large doses or for long-term therapy. Use with caution in Spleen and Stomach deficiency.

# Long Gu

*Os Draconis Fossilia*
*Sweet, astringent, slightly cold; Heart, Liver*

[Characteristics] It is the primary herb used as a heavy sedative to calm the spirit. Long Gu is a common herb used for conditions of heat disturbing upward with agitation, and Liver yang rising with dizziness and headache. Because of its astringent characteristic, it can also restrain leakage of the essence and used for patterns of unstable righteous qi with excessive sweating and spermatorrhea, etc.

## FUNCTIONS • INDICATIONS & MAJOR COMBINATIONS

**1. Sedate the Heart and calm the spirit:**
  - Agitation, palpitation or panic with palpitation and insomnia or seizures and manic behaviors. *+ Zhu Sha, Yuan Zhi*

**2. Pacify the Liver and subdue floating yang:**
  - Yin deficiency and yang ascending with irritability, bad temper, dizziness and vertigo. *+ Mu Li, Bai Shao*

**3. Astringe and restrain leakage of the essence:**
  - Spontaneous sweating or night sweating. *+ Mu Li, Wu Wei Zi*
  - Kidney deficiency with nocturnal emission. *+ Qian Shi, Sha Yuan Zi*
  - Unremitting Gushing and Leaking Syndromes. *+ Huang Qi, Bai Zhu*
  - Excessive or blood tinged vaginal discharge. *+ Hai Piao Xiao, Shan Yao*

**4. For sores with itchiness and discharge or chronic non-healing sores and ulcerations, apply the calcined and powdered form. This helps absorb dampness and accelerate the process of healing.**

[Dosage] 15-30 g. Crush and decoct first. Calcined form astringes and consolidates, and the raw form is used for other purposes.

[Comments] To sedate the Heart, calm the spirit, pacify the Liver, and subdue floating yang, Long Gu is usually combined with Mu Li. For differentiation and application (p. 189).

## [Addendum]
## Long Chi
### *Dens Draconis Fossilia*

Sweet, astringent and cool, it soothes and calms the mind; primarily used for irritability, palpitation, insomnia and dream-disturbed sleep. 15-30 g. Use the raw form or calcined form.

# Hu Po

*Succinum*
*Sweet, neutral; Heart, Liver, Bladder*

[Characteristics] Sweet and neutral, entering the Heart and Liver, or the blood level, it soothes and calms the mind, as well as invigorates the blood and dispels stasis. In addition, Hu Po enters the Bladder channel to promote urination and unblock the obstruction of the urinary tract.

| FUNCTIONS • INDICATIONS & MAJOR COMBINATIONS |
| --- |
| **1. Soothe and calm the spirit:**<br>• Convulsions, epilepsy and seizures. *+ Zhu Sha, Quan Xie*<br>• Palpitation, insomnia and dream-disturbed sleep. *+ Suan Zao Ren, Ye Jiao Teng* |
| **2. Invigorate the blood and expel stasis:**<br>• Blood stasis with amenorrhea. *+ San Leng, E Zhu* |
| **3. Promote urination and unblock the obstruction of the urinary passage:**<br>• Stone-type, Heat-type and especially Blood-type of Painful Urinary Dysfunctions. *+ Pu Huang* |

[Dosage] 1-3 g. To take this herb, add the powdered form into the strained decoction. Do not decoct.

# Suan Zao Ren

*Semen Ziziphi Spinosae*
*Sweet, sour, neutral; Heart, Liver, Gallbladder*

[Characteristics] Acting on the internal body, Suan Zao Ren's role is to tonify; while acting on the surface of the body, its role is to consolidate. Sweet and moist, Suan Zao Ren nourishes Heart yin and Liver blood to calm the mind. With its sour property, it astringes to stop deficient sweating. It is the imperial herb for nourishing the Heart, calming the mind, and astringing the deficient sweat.

**FUNCTIONS • INDICATIONS & MAJOR COMBINATIONS**

**1. Nourish the Heart and calm the spirit:**
- Heart and Liver blood deficiency with insomnia, panic with palpitation or unexplained palpitation. *+ Dang Gui, Bai Shao*
- Liver blood deficiency with insomnia. *+ Zhi Mu, Fu Ling*
- Heart and Kidney yin deficiency, or lack of communication between the Heart and Kidney with insomnia. *+ Bai Zi Ren, Yuan Zhi*

**2. Astringe abnormal sweating:**
- Spontaneous sweating and night sweating. *+ Dang Shen, Wu Wei Zi*

[Dosage] 10-20 g. or take the powdered form at bedtime, 1.5-3 g.

# Bai Zi Ren

*Semen Platycladi*
*Sweet, neutral; Heart, Kidney, Large Intestine*

[Characteristics] Sweet and moist to nourish, entering the Heart channel, Bai Zi Ren nourishes the Heart to calm the mind. It enters the Large Intestine channel to moisten the intestines and unblock the obstruction of bowel movements.

**FUNCTIONS • INDICATIONS & MAJOR COMBINATIONS**

**1. Nourish the Heart and calm the spirit:**
- Heart blood deficiency and malnourishment of the spirit with palpitation, insomnia and forgetfulness. *+ Ren Shen, Wu Wei Zi*

**2. Moisten the intestines and unblock the obstruction of bowel movements:**
- Injured body fluid and intestinal dryness with constipation. *+ Yu Li Ren, Xing Ren*

[Dosage] 10-20 g.

# Yuan Zhi

*Radix Polygalae*
*Acrid, bitter, slightly warm; Heart, Kidney, Lung*

[Characteristics] Yuan Zhi primarily enters the Heart and Kidney channels; it is the imperial herb for "communicating between the Heart and Kidney to soothe the mind". It is chiefly indicated for patterns of insomnia due to lack of communication between the Heart and Kidney. Because of its ability to dispel phlegm turbidity and open orifices, it is also used for disorientation due to phlegm obstructing orifice of the Heart.

| FUNCTIONS ● INDICATIONS & MAJOR COMBINATIONS |
| --- |
| **1. Soothe the Heart and calm the spirit:**<br>• Agitation or panic with palpitation. *+ Zhu Sha, Long Chi*<br>• Insufficiency of the yin and blood, or lack of communication between the Heart and Kidney with insomnia. *+ Suan Zao Ren, Bai Zi Ren*<br>• Heart and Spleen deficiency with insomnia. *+ Long Yan Rou, Fu Shen* |
| **2. Expel phlegm and open the orifices:**<br>• Turbid phlegm obstructing the Heart's orifice with emotional or mental confusion and disorientation. *+ Shi Chang Pu, Yu Jin*<br>• Coughing with copious sputum that is sticky and difficult to expectorate. *+ Xing Ren, Jie Geng* |
| **3. Reduce abscesses and swelling:**<br>• Swollen painful breast or toxic swelling such as sores, abscesses and boils. Take the powdered form with wine, or apply topically. |

[Dosage] 3-10 g.

[Precautions] It is not recommended for patients with peptic ulcer or gastritis.

**Herbs that Nourish the Heart and Calm the Spirit**

# He Huan Pi

*Cortex Albiziae*
*Sweet, neutral; Heart, Liver*

[Characteristics] Benefits the Heart and Spleen and relieves Liver constraint, as well as invigorates the blood to alleviate pain, generate tissue and mend fracture. It is commonly used for depression, irritability and insomnia due to emotional trauma, also for traumatic injuries, painful abscesses and swelling.

**FUNCTIONS • INDICATIONS & MAJOR COMBINATIONS**

### 1. Relieve Liver constraint and calm the spirit:
- Emotional trauma with short temper or depression, irritability, insomnia and poor memory. *+ Bai Zi Ren, Long Chi*

### 2. Invigorate the blood and reduce swelling:
- Traumatic injuries and bone fractures. *+ Dang Gui, Chuan Xiong*
- Lung abscess. *+ Bai Lian*
- Sores, abscesses and carbuncles. *+ Pu Gong Ying, Ye Ju Hua*

[Dosage] 10-15 g.

[Addendum]
## He Huan Hua
*Flos Albiziae*

Sweet and neutral, it has the effects of calming the mind and relieving the constraint; He Huan Hua is used for depression, irritability and agitation, forgetfulness and insomnia; it is commonly combined with herbs that calm the mind. 6-10 g.

## [Remarks & Differentiations]

### Zhu Sha — Ci Shi

| | Zhu Sha | Ci Shi |
|---|---|---|
| **C** | Heavy in quality, descend downward. Sedate the Heart and calm the spirit. | |
| **D** | • Mainly enters the Heart; strongly sedates the Heart and calms the spirit. <br><br> • Clears heat and relieves toxicity. | • Also enters the Liver and Kidney; can tonify the Liver and augment the Kidney. <br> • Improves visual and auditory acuities. <br> • Assists the Kidney to grasp the qi and calm wheezing. |

### Suan Zao Ren — Bai Zi Ren

| | Suan Zao Ren | Bai Zi Ren |
|---|---|---|
| **C** | Sweet in nature and moist in quality. Nourish the Heart and calm the spirit. Used for malnourishment of the Heart and spirit with insomnia. | |
| **D** | • Mainly enters the Liver and nourishes Liver blood. <br> • Astringes deficient sweat. | • Mainly enters the Heart and nourishes Heart blood. <br> • Moistens the intestines and unblocks the obstruction of bowel movements. |

# HERBS THAT
## Pacify the Liver and Extinguish Wind

With the primary functions of pacifying the Liver and extinguishing intenal wind, herbs in this category subdue Liver yang and stop tremors.

There are two subcategories. One contains herbs of mineral, metal and shell types that are heavy and descending to strongly suppress ascendant Liver yang. The other subcategory contains herbs that are made up of insects. The nature of these herbs is to search and gather up the wind from the collaterals. They are indicated for Liver yang rising with headache, irritability, short temper and red eyes, and for Liver wind swirling internally with dizziness, vertigo, convulsions, epilepsy and tremors.

With appropriate combinations, herbs in this category can be used for various conditions. For extreme heat generating wind, combine with herbs that clear heat and drain fire; for yin deficiency and yang rising with wind, add together herbs that nourish the yin and blood; in the case of yang rising and disturbing the mind, combine with herbs that calm the spirit.

Based on an individual herb's property, the use of warm and drying herbs for yin deficiency with yang rising is not recommended, as with the use of cool or cold herbs in chronic convulsion due to Spleen deficiency.

# Shi Jue Ming

*Concha Haliotidis*
*Salty, cold; Liver*

[Characteristics] Exclusively entering the Liver channel, Shi Jue Ming is an important herb that is salty and cold to clear Liver heat, and is heavy to subdue floating Liver yang. Additionally, by nourishing Liver yin, it can clear Liver heat and brighten the eyes. Combining with the appropriate herbs, it is indicated for dizziness due to Liver yang rising, and for ophthalmologic disorders due to Liver yin deficiency.

### FUNCTIONS • INDICATIONS & MAJOR COMBINATIONS

**1. Pacify the Liver and subdue the yang:**
- Liver yin deficiency and Liver yang rising with dizziness and vertigo. *+ Sheng Di Huang, Bai Shao*
- Ascendant Liver yang with headache, dizziness, vertigo, irritability and bad temper. *+ Xia Ku Cao, Gou Teng*

**2. Clear heat from the Liver and brighten the eyes:**
- Liver fire blazing up with red swollen painful eyes. *+ Jue Ming Zi, Ju Hua*
- Liver and Kidney yin deficiency with blurry vision. *+ Shu Di Huang, Tu Si Zi*
- Wind-heat with red eyes, pterygium or other superficial visual obstructions. *+ Mi Meng Hua, Gu Jing Cao*

[Dosage] 15-30 g. Crush and decoct first prior to adding in other herbs from the prescription.

[Comments] Both Shi Jue Ming and Cao Jue Ming share the functions of clearing heat from the Liver and brightening the eyes; these two herbs are commonly used for ophthalmologic disorders. The former, salty and heavy, cools Liver heat and anchors ascending Liver yang, as well as nourishes Liver yin, and it is mostly used for condition of yang rising. The latter, bitter and cold, strongly clears and drains Liver fire, is mostly used for exess fire in the Liver channel.

# Zhen Zhu Mu

*Concha Margaritifera*
*Salty, cold; Liver, Heart*

[Characteristics] Heavy quality, it enters the Liver and Heart channels. It clears heat from the Liver and Heart, pacifies the Liver and subdues floating yang, and sedates the Heart and calms the spirit. It can also brighten the eyes. Zhen Zhu Mu is indicated for dizziness, vertigo, irritability and insomnia due to Liver yang rising, and for red eyes due to Liver fire blazing upward.

| FUNCTIONS • INDICATIONS & MAJOR COMBINATIONS |
|---|
| **1. Pacify the Liver, subdue the yang, sedate the Heart and calm the spirit:** <br> • Insufficient Liver yin and ascendant Liver yang with headache, dizziness and vertigo. *+ Bai Shao, Sheng Di Huang* <br> • Ascendant Liver yang disturbing upward with irritability, insomnia and restlessness. *+ Long Gu, Mu Li* <br> • Malnourishment of the Heart and mind with insomnia, dream-disturbed sleep and forgetfulness. *+ Suan Zao Ren, Long Yan Rou* |
| **2. Clear heat from the Liver and brighten the eyes:** <br> • Liver fire blazing up with red swollen painful eyes. *+ Shi Jue Ming, Ju Hua* <br> • Liver deficiency with dull or blurry vision. *+ Cang Zhu* |
| **3. For skin disorders due to dampness with itchiness, apply the powdered form topically.** |

[Dosage] 15-30 g. Crush and decoct first before adding other herbs in the prescription.

# Mu Li

*Concha Ostreae*
*Salty, astringent, slightly cold; Liver, Kidney*

[Characteristics] Heavy to descend, it has a very strong effect on pacifying the Liver and subduing the yang. Additionally, it nourishes the yin and clears heat, and is primarily used for wind swirling internally due to yin deficiency and yang rising. Mu Li is salty to soften hardness and dissipate nodules, and is used for scrofula and goiter. It is also astringent to restrain, and used for treating leakage patterns of the essence.

### FUNCTIONS • INDICATIONS & MAJOR COMBINATIONS

**1. Pacify the Liver and subdue the yang:**
- Yin deficiency and ascendant yang with dizziness, vertigo, tinnitus, headaches, irritability and insomnia. *+ Long Gu, Gui Ban*
- Extreme heat injuring the yin and generating internal wind with spasms and contractions of the limbs. *+ Gui Ban, Bie Jia*

**2. Soften hardness and dissipate nodules:**
- Phlegm-fire complex with lumps around the neck such as scrofula and goiter. *+ Zhe Bei Mu, Xuan Shen*
- *Zheng Jia Ji Ju. + Dan Shen, Bie Jia*

**3. Astringe and restrain the leakage of essence:**
- Spontaneous sweating or night sweating. *+ Ma Huang Gen*
- Kidney deficiency with nocturnal emission and spermatorrhea. *+ Sha Yuan Zi, Qian Shi*
- Gushing and Leaking Syndromes or excessive vaginal discharge. *+ Hai Piao Xiao, Shan Yao*

**4. Control acidity for sour regurgitation and stomach upset.**

[Dosage] 15-30 g. Decoct first. Calcined form to astringe and bind; raw for other purposes.

[Comments] Both Mu Li and Long Gu are heavy substances that share similar functions; therefore, they are usually combined together for mutual reinforcement. Long Gu mainly enters the Heart channel to strongly sedate the Heart and calm the spirit for agitation, palpitation, insomnia, panic and mania. Mainly entering the Liver channel, Mu Li has an added effect to nourish the yin at the same time, strongly subdues the yang; therefore, it is indicated for both deficient and excess patterns of wind swirling internally. It can also soften hardness and dissipate nodules for lumps around the neck.

**Herbs that Pacify the Liver and Subdue the Yang**

# Dai Zhe Shi

*Haematitum*
*Bitter, cold; Liver, Heart*

[Characteristics] A bitter and cold herb, it clears Liver fire and subdues Liver yang. It is a common herb used for Liver fire blazing upward and Liver yang rising. As a heavy substance, Dai Zhe Shi descends the rebellious qi of Lung and Stomach to treat coughing, wheezing, hiccup or vomiting. Additionally, it cools the blood and stops bleeding for the treatment of hemorraging due to heat causing reckless movement of the blood.

**FUNCTIONS • INDICATIONS & MAJOR COMBINATIONS**

**1. Pacify the Liver and subdue the yang:**
- Ascendant Liver yang with dizziness, vertigo, headaches, irritability and insomnia. *+ Long Gu, Mu Li*

**2. Redirect rebellious qi downward:**
- Rebellious Stomach qi with belching, hiccup, nausea and vomiting. *+ Xuan Fu Hua, Ban Xia*
- Lung and Kidney deficiency with shortness of breath, wheezing and requiring sitting upright to breath. *+ Dang Shen, Shan Zhu Yu*

**3. Cool the blood and stop bleeding:**
- Heat in the blood with hematemesis, subcutaneous and mucosa bleeding. *+ Bai Shao, Zhu Ru*
- Heat in the blood with Gushing and Leaking Syndromes. *+ Chi Shi Zhi, Wu Ling Zhi*

[Dosage] 15-30 g. crush and decoct first before adding in other herbs from the formula. 1-3 g. if making pill form. Raw herb can pacify the Liver and redirect rebellious qi downward; calcine to stop bleeding.

[Precautions] Contraindicated during pregnancy.

**Herbs that Pacify the Liver and Subdue the Yang**

# Ling Yang Jiao

*Cornu Saigae Tataricae*
*Salty, cold; Liver, Heart*

**[Characteristics]** It is cold to clear heat and salty to enter the blood level. Entering the Liver channel, Ling Yang Jiao is the primary herb for extreme heat generating wind with convulsions, epilepsy and seizures or contractions of the extremities. It has additional effects of clearing heat, draining fire and relieving toxicity.

**FUNCTIONS • INDICATIONS & MAJOR COMBINATIONS**

**1. Extinguish wind and stop tremors:**
- Intractable high fever generating internal wind with convulsions, epilepsy and seizures, contractions and spasms. *+ Gou Teng, Ju Hua*

**2. Clear heat from the Liver and brighten the eyes:**
- Ascendant Liver yang with blurry vision. *+ Shi Jue Ming, Ju Hua*
- Liver fire blazing up with red eyes. *+ Jue Ming Zi, Huang Qin*

**3. Clear heat and relieve toxicity:**
- Warm-Febrile Disease with high fever, delirium, loss of consciousness, contractions and spasms. *+ Shi Gao, Han Shui Shi*

**[Dosage]** 1-3 g. requiring decoction of this herb alone for a minimum of two hours, or use 0.3-0.5 g. if filing it to powder.

**[Comments]** Both Ling Yang Jiao and Xi Jiao are salty and cold herbs that enter the Heart and Liver, or blood level. In the cases of heat entering the nutritive and blood level of Warm-Febrile Disease with delirium, loss of consciousness, convulsions and contractions, these two herbs are usually combined together. Ling Yang Jiao mainly enters the Liver channel to drain Liver fire and extinguish Liver wind; it is usually not the herb of choice for patient who presents with only loss of consciousness. Xi Jiao, on the contrary, mainly enters the Heart channel to clear heat from the Heart and cool the blood; it is usually the herb of choice in the treatment for delirious comatose resulting from heat entering the Heart, or nutritive level.

**[Addendum]**
### Shan Yang Jiao
*Cornu Naemorhedus Goral*

Salty and cold, it enters the Liver channel to pacify the Liver and control convulsions. It is used for convulsions and contractions due to Liver fire blazing up or Liver yang rising. In modern application, it is used in place of Ling Yang Jiao at a larger dose of 10-15 g. Refer to Ling Yang Jiao for application methods.

# Tian Ma

*Rhizoma Gastrodiae*
*Sweet, neutral; Liver*

[Characteristics] Sweet, neutral, soft and moist, it only enters the Liver channel. Tian Ma nourishes the yin, pacifies the Liver, extinguishes wind and stops tremors. It is also known as "Ding Feng Cao", herb that arrests wind; therefore, it is the imperial herb for the treatment of wind. With the appropriate combinations, it is indicated for all patterns of Liver wind swirling internally regardless of heat or cold and deficiency or excess. Additionally, it dispels external wind, unblocks the channels and alleviates painful obstruction.

| FUNCTIONS • INDICATIONS & MAJOR COMBINATIONS |
|---|
| **1. Extinguish wind and stop tremors:** |
| • Acute childhood convulsion. *+ Gou Teng, Ling Yang Jiao* |
| • Chronic childhood convulsion. *+ Ren Shen, Bai Zhu* |
| • Tetanus, contractions, spasms, epilepsy, seizures and opisthotonos. *+ Tian Nan Xing, Bai Fu Zi* |
| **2. Pacify the Liver and subdue the yang:** |
| • Ascendant yang with dizziness, vertigo and headaches. *+ Gou Teng, Huang Qin* |
| • Wind-phlegm disturbing up with nausea and dizziness. *+ Ban Xia, Bai Zhu* |
| • Stubborn migraine headaches. *+ Chuan Xiong* |
| **3. Expel wind and unblock obstruction in the collaterals:** |
| • Wind-dampness Painful Obstruction with numbness and paralysis of the extremities. *+ Qin Jiao, Sang Ji Sheng* |

[Dosage] 3-10 g. 1-1.5 g. when using powdered form.

[Comments] As the imperial herb for treating wind, Tian Ma is widely used for Liver wind swirling internally with dizziness and vertigo. However, if dizziness and vertigo are accompanied by heavy sensation of the head, nausea and vomiting, and white greasy tongue coating, there must be Spleen deficiency involved to generate phlegm. This dizziness and vertigo require the combination of Tian Ma and Ban Xia, the classic pair for dizziness and vertigo due to wind-phlegm complex. While Ban Xia dries dampness and transforms phlegm, descends rebellious qi and stops vomiting, Tian Ma extinguishes wind and alleviates dizziness and vertigo.

# Gou Teng

*Ramulus Uncariae cum Uncis*
*Sweet, slightly cold; Liver, Pericardium*

**[Characteristics]** Sweet and slightly cold, it clears heat as well as pacifies the Liver to extinguish wind. Gou Teng is a common herb for extreme heat generating wind, and Liver yang rising.

FUNCTIONS • INDICATIONS & MAJOR COMBINATIONS

**1. Extinguish wind and stop tremors:**
- Extreme heat generating wind in Warm-Febrile Disease with contractions and spasms of the limbs. *+ Ling Yang Jiao, Ju Hua*
- Acute childhood convulsion with high fever. *+ Tian Ma, Quan Xie*

**2. Clear heat and pacify the Liver:**
- Liver excess heat with headaches. *+ Xia Ku Cao, Huang Qin*
- Ascendant Liver yang with headaches. *+ Shi Jue Ming, Ju Hua*

**[Dosage]** 10-15 g. add to the decoction towards the end.

# Ci Ji Li

*Fructus Tribuli*
*Bitter, acrid, neutral; Liver*

**[Characteristics]** Light in quality and acrid in nature, it disperses; it is also bitter to descend. Ci Ji Li pacifies the Liver and extinguishes wind, as well as disperses wind-heat from the Liver channel, and spreads the constrained Liver qi.

FUNCTIONS • INDICATIONS & MAJOR COMBINATIONS

**1. Pacify the Liver and facilitate the smooth flow of Liver qi:**
- Ascendant Liver yang with headaches, dizziness and vertigo. *+ Gou Teng, Zhen Zhu Mu*
- Constrained Liver qi with distention in the chest and hypochondriac regions. *+ Chai Hu, Qing Pi*

**2. Dispel wind and brighten the eyes:**
- Wind-heat attacking up with red teary eyes. *+ Ju Hua, Jue Ming Zi*
- Wind rash with significant itching. *+ Chan Tui, Jing Jie*

**[Dosage]** 6-10 g.

**[Comments]** The alternative name is Bai Ji Li.

# Quan Xie

*Scorpio*
*Acrid, neutral, toxic; Liver*

[Characteristics] Exclusively entering the Liver channel to extinguish wind, Quan Xie is neutral and is indicated for all patterns of wind. In addition, the nature of this herb is to search and gather up the wind to unblock obstruction in the collaterals for Wind-dampness Painful Obstruction and stubborn headache. With topical application, it relieves toxicity, dissipates nodules and alleviates pain.

| FUNCTIONS • INDICATIONS & MAJOR COMBINATIONS |
|---|

**1. Extinguish wind and stop tremors:**
- Spasms and contractions resulting from various pathogenesis. Use the powdered form. *+ Wu Gong*
- Acute childhood convulsion. *+ Tian Ma, Gou Teng*
- Spleen deficiency causing chronic childhood convulsion. *+ Dang Shen, Bai Zhu*
- Wind stroke with facial paralysis. *+ Bai Fu Zi, Bai Jiang Can*
- Tetanus. *+ Dan Nan Xing, Chan Tui*

**2. Unblock obstruction in the collaterals and alleviate pain:**
- Wind-cold-damp Painful Obstruction with spasm of the sinews or deformed joints. Use this herb alone in powdered form, or *+ Chuan Wu, Bai Hua She*
- Stubborn headaches. *+ Wu Gong, Bai Jiang Can*

**3. Relieve toxicity and dissipate nodules:**
- Toxic sores, abscesses and carbuncles, commonly combined with other herbs to make plaster for topical application. *+ Wu Gong, Zhi Zi*

[Dosage] 3-5 g. Reduce to 0.6-1 g when using powdered form. Do not exceed the recommended dosage because of its toxic nature.

[Precautions] Contraindicated during pregnancy.

[Comments] ❶ The alternative name is Quan Chong

❷ The tail of Quan Xie has the strongest effect. According to ancient documentation, "The therapeutic strength is located in its tail."

# Wu Gong

*Scolopendra*
*Acrid, warm, toxic; Liver*

[Characteristics] Having similar but stronger effects compared to Quan Xie, Wu Gong and Quan Xie are used together in clinical applications.

## FUNCTIONS • INDICATIONS & MAJOR COMBINATIONS

### 1. Extinguish wind and stop tremors:
- Spasms and contractions resulting from various pathogenesis. Use the powdered form *+ Quan Xie*
- Acute childhood convulsion. *+ Bai Jiang Can, Gou Teng*
- Wind stroke with facial paralysis. *+ Bai Fu Zi, Bai Jiang Can*

### 2. Unblock obstruction in the collaterals and alleviate pain:
- Stubborn Wind-damp Painful Obstruction. *+ Wei Ling Xian, Fang Feng*
- Stubborn headaches. *+ Quan Xie, Bai Jiang Can*

### 3. Relieve toxicity and dissipate nodules:
- Toxic sores, abscesses and carbuncles, commonly combined with other herbs to make plaster for topical application. *+ Quan Xie*
- For perforated scrofula with discharge, apply the powdered form.
- Poison snakebite. *+ Huang Lian, Da Huang*

[Dosage] 1-3 g. Reduce to 0.6-1 g when using powdered form. Do not exceed the recommended dosage because of its toxic nature.

[Precautions] Contraindicated during pregnancy.

# Bai Jiang Can

*Bombyx Batryticatus*
*Salty, acrid, neutral; Liver, Lung*

[Characteristics] Acrid to dispel wind, salty to soften hardness, dissipate nodules and resolve phlegm, Bai Jiang Can extinguishes internal Liver wind, as well as dispels external wind-heat. It is primarily indicated for acute or chronic childhood convulsion, wind-heat with headaches or red eyes, and for goiter and scrofula.

| FUNCTIONS • INDICATIONS & MAJOR COMBINATIONS |
|---|
| **1. Extinguish wind, resolve phlegm and stop tremors:** |
| • Acute childhood convulsion due to phlegm-heat. *+ Dan Nan Xing, Niu Huang* |
| • Chronic childhood convulsion. *+ Dang Shen, Bai Zhu* |
| • Wind stroke with facial paralysis. *+ Quan Xie, Bai Fu Zi* |
| • Tetanus. *+ Quan Xie, Wu Gong* |
| **2. Dispel wind-heat:** |
| • Wind-heat with headaches and red eyes. *+ Sang Ye, Ju Hua* |
| • Wind-heat attacking above with swollen sore throat. *+ Jie Geng, Gan Cao* |
| • Wind rash with skin itchiness. *+ Chan Tui, Bo He* |
| **3. Relieve toxicity and dissipate nodules:** |
| • Phlegm accumulating with scrofula. *+ Xia Ku Cao, Zhe Bei Mu* |

[Dosage] 3-10 g. Reduce to 1-1.5 g when using powdered form. Raw for dispersing wind-heat; fried form for other purposes.

[Comments] The alternative names are Jiang Can and Tian Chong.

# Di Long

*Pheretima*
***Salty, cold; Liver, Spleen, Bladder***

[Characteristics] Salty and cold, Di Long descends and drains downward with a strong migrating ability. Di Long enters the Liver channel to clear Liver heat, extinguish wind and control convulsions; it also unblocks obstructions in the collaterals to alleviate pain. It enters the Lung channel to clear Lung heat and calm wheezing. It enters the Kidney channel to facilitate the flow in the water passage and unblock the obstruction of the urinary tract.

### FUNCTIONS • INDICATIONS & MAJOR COMBINATIONS

#### 1. Clear heat and extinguish wind:
- Extreme heat generating internal wind in Warm-Febrile Disease with delirium and loss of consciousness. *+ Gou Teng, Niu Huang*
- Pediatric convulsion with high fever, spasms and contractions of the limbs. *+ Zhu Sha*

#### 2. Unblock the collaterals:
- Painful obstruction with limited range of motion of the extremities.
  — Heat-type of Painful Obstruction. *+ Sang Zhi, Ren Dong Teng*
  — Cold-dampness Painful Obstruction. *+ Chuan Wu, Cao Wu*
  — Hemiplegia status post wind stroke. *+ Huang Qi, Dang Gui Wei*

#### 3. Calm wheezing:
- Heat accumulated in the Lung with asthma and copious sputum. *+Shi Gao, Ma Huang*

#### 4. Promote urination:
- Heat accumulated in the Bladder with dysuria. *+ Che Qian Zi, Mu Tong*

[Dosage] 6-15 g. 10-20 g. when using the fresh herb. 1-2 g. when using powdered form.

[Comments] ❶ The alternative name is Qiu Yin.

❷ Di Long has a good therapeutic effect for decreasing blood pressure related to Liver yang rising when taken orally.

## [Remarks & Differentiations]

### Shi Jue Ming — Zhen Zhu Mu

|   | Shi Jue Ming | Zhen Zhu Mu |
|---|---|---|
| C | Pacify the Liver and subdue floating yang. Clear heat from the Liver and brighten the eyes. | |
| D | • Enters the Liver channel only. | • Enters the Liver and Heart channels, settles the Heart and calms the spirit for ascendant yang disturbing upward with insomnia and agitation. |

### Tian Ma — Gou Teng

|   | Tian Ma | Gou Teng |
|---|---|---|
| C | Extinguish wind and stop tremors. Combined for mutual reinforcement for Liver wind swirling internally with contractions and tremors. | |
| D | • Sweet, neutral, soft and moist to nourish the yin.<br>• Treats both internal and external wind. | • Sweet and slightly cold to clear heat.<br>• Primarily used for extreme heat generating internal wind. |

# HERBS THAT
## Open the Orifices                                15

Opening up the sensory orifices and awakening the spirit are their primary functions. The majority of herbs from this group are acrid to disperse, warm to open up the orifices and aromatic to migrate, and they enter the Heart channel. These herbs are very effective for treating loss of consciousness and delirium due to heat trapped in the Pericardium or turbid-phlegm obstructing Heart's orifice, and also for convulsions, epilepsy, seizures or wind-stroke with sudden loss of consciousness.

Loss of consciousness can be divided into excess or deficiency. For deficient pattern, also known as abandoned disorder, the treatment principle should be to tonify the qi to rescue the collapse. Herbs from this chapter are used in excess patterns only. Excess pattern, also known as closed disorder, have two types, heat or cold. For those of heat-type closed disorder, herbs that cool and open the orifices should be selected with herbs that clear heat and relieve toxicity. For those of cold-type closed disorder, herbs that warm and open the orifices should be used and combined with herbs that expel cold and regulate the qi.

Herbs that open the orifices are used only in emergency cases and should be for temporary use. They are contraindicated for abandoned disorder. These herbs are mostly prepared in pill or powered forms because its acrid and dispersing nature evaporates quickly if prepared in decoction.

# She Xiang

*Moschus*
*Acrid, warm; Heart, Spleen*

[Characteristics] In addition to its acrid and dispersing properties, She Xiang is also aromatic and has a strong migrating ability. Entering the Heart channel, it is the imperial herb to open up sensory orifices and awaken the spirit. It is the first choice for comatose patients classified as closed disorders regardless of cold or heat types. She Xiang also enters the blood level to invigorate the blood and transform stasis, reduce swelling and alleviate pain. It is an effective herb for pain related to blood stasis, swelling and pain related to sores and abscesses.

## FUNCTIONS • INDICATIONS & MAJOR COMBINATIONS

**1. Open the orifices and revive the spirit:**
  - Heat-type of closed disorder, in which the warm pathogenic factors cover the orifices causing delirium, coma, contractions, convulsions and spasms, and phlegm-heat obstructing the orifices and meridians accompanied with wind stroke. *+ Xi Jiao, Ling Yang Jiao*
  - Cold-type of closed disorder, in which cold-phlegm and turbid damp-ness cover the orifices manifesting with disorientation or coma. *+ Su He Xiang, Ding Xiang*

**2. Invigorate the blood, transform blood stasis and alleviate pain:**
  - Blood stasis with amenorrhea. *+ Tao Ren, Hong Hua*
  - Traumatic injuries with hematoma and swelling. *+ Ru Xiang, Mo Yao*
  - Blood stasis causing headaches. *+ Tao Ren, Lao Cong*
  - Chest Painful Obstruction. *+ Tao Ren, Mu Xiang*
  - *Zheng Jia Ji Ju.* *+ E Zhu, Hong Hua*

**3. Dissipate nodules and reduce swelling:**
  - Toxic sores, abscesses and carbuncles. *+ Xiong Huang, Ru Xiang*
  - Swollen sore throat and sores in the mouth and tongue. *+ Bing Pian, Niu Huang*

**4. To induce delivery, facilitate the passage of a stillbirth delivery, or de-scend the placenta.** *+ Rou Gui*

[Dosage] 0.06-0.1 g. Do not decoct, to be taken in pill or powdered forms only.

[Precautions] Contraindicated during pregnancy.

# Niu Huang

*Calculus Bovis*
*Bitter, cool; Heart, Liver*

**[Characteristics]** A bitter, cool and aromatic substance, it enters the Heart channel to clear heat, open the orifices and transform phlegm. It enters the Liver channel to cool the Liver, extinguish wind and control convulsions. Niu Huang is the imperial herb to resolve phlegm and open the orifices, to arrest wind and stop tremors.

**FUNCTIONS • INDICATIONS & MAJOR COMBINATIONS**

**1. Transform phlegm and open the orifices:**
- Phlegm-heat obstructing Heart's orifice with delirium or coma, and phlegm-heat obstructing the meridians causing wind stroke with hemiplegia. *+ She Xiang*

**2. Extinguish wind and stop tremors:**
- Extreme heat generating internal wind. *+ Zhu Sha, Quan Xie*

**3. Clear heat and relieve toxicity:**
- Swollen sore throat or sores in the mouth and tongue. *+ Zhen Zhu*
- Toxic sores, abscesses and carbuncles. *+ Da Huang, Huang Qin*
- Breast abscess and scrofula. *+ She Xiang, Mo Yao*

**[Dosage]** 0.2-0.5 g. Do not decoct, to be taken in pill or powdered forms only.

**[Precautions]** Contraindicated during pregnancy.

**[Comments]** Niu Huang, She Xiang, Xi Jiao and Ling Yang Jiao are commonly combined for Warm-Febrile Disease with comatose. Individual differences are:

**She Xiang**, with the aromatic nature and strong migrating ability, is the first choice from this group of herbs to open up the orifices and awaken the spirit in both cold or heat type of closed disorders.

**Niu Huang** is relatively more effective in clearing heat from the Heart and transforming phlegm to open up the orifices. It is indicated for phlegm-heat obstructing Heart's orifice. It can also extinguish wind and stop tremors.

**Xi Jiao** mainly enters the Heart channel. Its primary functions are to clear heat from the Heart and cool the blood. It is indicated for heat entering the nutritive and blood levels in Warm-Febrile Disease with high fever and coma.

**Ling Yang Jiao**, mainly entering the Liver channel, has good effects on draining Liver fire and extinguishing Liver wind. In the conditions of comatose due to heat lodged in Heart's orifice with convulsions, epilepsy, contractions and spasms, Ling Yang Jiao is added.

# Bing Pian

*Borneolum Syntheticum*
*Acrid, bitter, slightly cold; Heart, Spleen, Lung*

[Characteristics] Clears heat from the Heart and opens the orifices; it has mild effect in treating comatose patients classified as heat-type of closed disorder. Bing Pian can also be applied topically to clear heat, alleviate pain and generate the tissue as a common herb for sores and swelling, and ear-nose-throat disorders.

**FUNCTIONS • INDICATIONS & MAJOR COMBINATIONS**

**1. Open the orifices and revive the spirit:**
- Warm-Febrile Disease with comatose. *+ She Xiang, Xi Jiao*

**2. Alleviate pain and generate the tissue:**
- Red swollen painful eyes. Use alone as eye drops.
- Swollen sore throat or sores in the mouth and tongue.
- Non-healing sores and ulcers. *+ Ru Xiang, Xue Jie*

[Dosage] 0.03-0.1 g. Do not decoct, to be taken in pill or powdered forms only.

[Precautions] Contraindicated during pregnancy.

# Su He Xiang

*Styrax*
*Acrid, warm; Heart, Spleen*

[Characteristics] Acrid and dispersing, warm and unblocking, with a strong aromatic fragrant, Su He Xiang is primarily used for comatose patients classified as cold-type of closed disorder. It also disperses cold to alleviate pain.

**FUNCTIONS • INDICATIONS & MAJOR COMBINATIONS**

**1. Open the orifices and revive the spirit:**
- Cold-phlegm and turbid dampness obstructed internally accompanied with wind stroke, and cold-type of closed disorder. *+ She Xiang*

**2. Dispel cold and alleviate pain:**
- Chest Painful Obstruction. *+ Bing Pian, Tan Xiang*
- Cold congealing and qi stagnation with distention and pain in the chest and abdomen. *+ Wu Yao, Yan Hu Suo*

[Dosage] 0.3-1 g. Do not decoct, to be taken in pill or powdered forms only.

[Precautions] Contraindicated during pregnancy.

# Shi Chang Pu

*Rhizoma Acori Tatarinowii*
*Acrid, warm; Heart, Stomach*

[Characteristics] Acrid to disperse, warm to unblock, and aromatic to transform dampness and to migrate, Shi Chang Pu transforms phlegm, opens up the orifices and awakens the spirit. It also transforms dampness and harmonizes the Stomach. It is used for comatose due to phlegm-dampness obstructing Heart's orifice, and for stifling sensation in the chest due to dampness accumulating in the middle burner.

| FUNCTIONS • INDICATIONS & MAJOR COMBINATIONS |
| --- |
| **1. Open up the orifices and quiet the spirit:**<br>• Phlegm-dampness obstructing Heart's orifice with disorientation and loss of consciousness. *+ Yu Jin, Ban Xia*<br>• Phlegm-heat with seizures. *+ Huang Lian, Zhu Ru*<br>• Phlegm obstructing the orifices with deafness. *+ Yuan Zhi, Fu Ling* |
| **2. Transform dampness and harmonize the Stomach:**<br>• Dampness accumulated in the middle burner with nausea, stifling sensation in the chest and greasy tongue coating. *+ Huo Xiang, Cang Zhu*<br>• Dysentery disorder due to heat toxins. *+ Huang Lian, Chen Pi* |

[Dosage] 6-10 g.

# HERBS THAT

## Tonify 16

Herbs in this category aim towards strengthening the deficiency by replenishing the vital substances and strengthening physical capabilities to enhance the defensive mechanism against pathogenic influences and improve the conditions of weakness.

There are four subcategories of tonics: (1) herbs that tonify the qi, (2) herbs that tonify the blood, (3) herbs that tonify the yin, and (4) herbs that tonify the yang. They are ued to treat all patterns of deficiency, such as Spleen and Lung qi deficiency, Heart and Liver blood deficiency, Lung and Stomach yin deficiency, Liver and Kidney yin deficiency or Spleen and Kidney yang deficiency.

The vital substances, qi, blood, yin and yang, are inter-dependent to each other physiologically. They also inter-influence each other during pathological situations. Therefore, the tonics from different subcategories are usually combined together to enhance the therapeutic effects. These herbs are not to be used in excess conditions. However, in coexistence of pathogenic influences with deficient righteous qi, tonics should be combined with herbs that expel pathogenic influences to support the righteous qi to expel the pathogenic factors.

When using tonics, especially those with cloying natures, combining with herbs that strengthen the Spleen is recommended.

# Ren Shen

*Radix Ginseng*
*Sweet, slightly bitter, slightly warm; Spleen, Lung*

[Characteristics] Ren Shen is characterized by its ability to strongly tonify basal qi. In critical and acute conditions, it rescues the collapsed qi; in chronic conditions, Ren Shen tonifies the deficiency. It is the imperial herb for extreme collapse of basal qi and consumptive deficiency. It also strengthens the Spleen and tonifies the Lung. Moreover, it generates the fluid, benefits Heart qi and calms the spirit.

| FUNCTIONS • INDICATIONS & MAJOR COMBINATIONS |
| --- |

**1. Strongly tonify basal qi:**
- For extreme collapsed qi or abandoned conditions due to severe loss of blood, excessive diarrhea, sweating and vomiting with pale complexion, profuse sweating, shallow respiration and minute pulse, this herb is used alone, called "Du Shen Tang".
- Collapsed qi and devastated yang with profuse sweating, icy-cold extremities and shortness of breath. *+ Fu Zi*

**2. Strengthen the Spleen and tonify the Lung:**
- Spleen and Stomach qi deficiency with fatigue, lack of appetite, abdominal distention and loose stool. *+ Bai Zhu, Fu Ling*
- Lung qi deficiency or the Kidney fails to grasp the qi with breathlessness and wheezing, exacerbation on exertion. *+ Ge Jie, Hu Tao Rou*

**3. Generate the fluid by tonifying the qi:**
- Qi and yin deficiency with shortness of breath, spontaneous sweating, thirst and minute pulse. *+ Mai Men Dong, Wu Wei Zi*

**4. Benefit Heart qi and calm the spirit:**
- Qi and blood deficiency with insomnia. *+ Dang Gui, Long Yan Rou*

[Dosage] 3-10 g. simmer separately for a long time, then add to the strained decoction of other herbs in the prescription. 1-2 g if using powdered form. Increase dose to 15-30 g for abandoned conditions.

[Precautions] Incompatible with Li Lu, antagonized with Wu Ling Zhi. Avoid taking turnips while on this herb as turnips could reduce the effects of Ren Shen.

[Comments] ❶ The wild grown species, known as Ye Shan Shen, has a stronger tonifying effect compared to the cultivated type, Yuan Yi Shen.

❷ With the various processes of Yuan Yi Shen, there are also Bai Shen, Hong Shen and Sheng Shai Shen, each with slightly different effects.

# Dang Shen

*Radix Codonopsis*
*Sweet, neutral; Spleen, Lung*

[Characteristics] Dang Shen is characterized by its ability to tonify Spleen and Stomach qi. It has similar functions as Ren Shen, however, less effective. Dang Shen, a common herb for deficiency of Spleen and Lung qi, essence and blood, can be used in place of Ren Shen for most prescriptions except for critical situation of qi collapse.

| FUNCTIONS • INDICATIONS & MAJOR COMBINATIONS |
|---|
| **1. Strengthen the Spleen and tonify the Lung:** |
| • Spleen and Stomach qi deficiency with fatigue, lack of appetite, abdominal distention and loose stool. *+ Bai Zhu, Fu Ling* |
| • Prolapsed Disorder due to sunken Spleen qi with chronic diarrhea and prolapse of organs. *+ Huang Qi, Sheng Ma* |
| • Lung qi deficiency with shortness of breath, cough, wheezing, weak and low voice. *+ Huang Qi, Wu Wei Zi* |
| **2. Generate the fluid and nourish the blood:** |
| • Qi and yin deficiency with shortness of breath, spontaneous sweating and thirst. *+ Mai Men Dong, Wu Wei Zi* |
| • Heat injuring the qi and yin in recovery stage of Warm-Febrile Disease with fever, irritability and thirst. *+ Shi Gao, Zhu Ye* |
| • Qi and blood deficiency with weakness, lassitude, dizziness and palpitation. *+ Dang Gui, Shu Di Huang* |

[Dosage] 10-20 g. Increase the dose when used in place of Ren Shen.

[Precautions] Incompatible with Li Lu.

[Comments] Dang Shen and Ren Shen were recognized as one entity in ancient time until the formation of the book, <u>Ben Cao Cong Xin</u> (Qing Dynasty, AC1757). As a result, Dang Shen is currently used in place of Ren Shen when formulating ancient prescriptions. Dang Shen is used for chronic and mild qi deficiency while Ren Shen is used for severe collapsed qi and devastated yang.

**Herbs that Tonify the Qi**

# Tai Zi Shen

*Radix Pseudostellariae*
*Sweet, slightly bitter, neutral; Spleen, Lung*

[Characteristics] Mildly tonifies the qi. Tai Zi Shen tonifies Spleen and Lung qi, and nourishes the yin to generate the fluid. It is used in conditions of Spleen and Lung qi deficiency accompanied by yin deficiency.

**FUNCTIONS • INDICATIONS & MAJOR COMBINATIONS**

**Strengthen the Spleen, augment the qi and generate the fluid:**
- Spleen deficiency with poor appetite and fatigue. *+ Shan Yao*
- Qi and blood deficiency with sweating and palpitation. *+ Wu Wei Zi*

[Dosage] 15-30 g.

[Precautions] Incompatible with Li Lu.

[Comments] ❶ The alternative name is Hai Er Shen.

❷ In ancient herbal documentation, Tai Zi Shen was the smaller variety of Ren Shen, from the family of Panax. The Tai Zi Shen used today is from the family of Pseudostellaria.

# Xi Yang Shen

*Radix Panacis Quinquefolii*
*Sweet, slightly bitter, cold; Heart, Lung, Kidney*

[Characteristics] Sweet and cold, benefits the qi and nourishes the yin; bitter and cold, clears heat or fire. It is used in deficiency of qi and yin with deficient heat.

**FUNCTIONS • INDICATIONS & MAJOR COMBINATIONS**

**Tonify the qi, nourish the yin and clear heat:**
- Qi and yin deficiency after febrile disease with irritability, thirst and weakness. *+ Sheng Di Huang, Mai Men Dong*
- Yin deficiency with empty fire causing dry cough, scanty sputum or blood-tinged sputum. *+ Mai Men Dong, Zhi Mu*
- For yin deficiency with dry throat and thirst, used alone in decoction.

[Dosage] 3-6 g. Simmer separately for a long time before adding into the strained decoction of other herbs in the prescription.

[Precautions] Incompatible with Li Lu.

[Comments] Categorized into the herbs that tonify the yin in some textbooks.

# Huang Qi

*Radix Astragali*
*Sweet, slightly warm; Spleen, Lung*

[Characteristics] Strengthens the Spleen and tonifies the Lung. Characterized by raising yang qi, it is the imperial herb for treating sunken Spleen qi. It consolidates the surface and augments protective qi to stop spontaneous sweating. It tonifies righteous qi to promote the discharge of pus, and generates the tissue for non-healing ulcers and sores due to qi and blood deficiency. As a strong qi tonic, it is often used in conditions of qi and blood deficiency, qi deficiency with blood stasis, and edema due to Spleen qi deficiency.

| FUNCTIONS • INDICATIONS & MAJOR COMBINATIONS |
|---|
| **1. Tonify the qi and raise the yang:**<br>• Prolapse Disorder due to sunken Spleen qi with chronic diarrhea and prolapse of organs. *+ Sheng Ma, Chai Hu*<br>• Failure to control blood due to qi deficiency with bloody stool, Gushing and Leaking Syndromes. *+ Ren Shen, Dang Gui*<br>• Blood deficiency due to qi deficiency with low grade fever, irritability and forceless flooding pulse. *+ Dang Gui* |
| **2. Augment protective qi and consolidate the surface:**<br>• Qi deficiency with spontaneous sweating and recurrent colds. *+ Bai Zhu, Fang Feng* |
| **3. Promote the discharge of pus and the generation of tissue:**<br>• Non-healing ulcers and sores or non-perforated abscesses due to qi and blood deficiency. *+ Rou Gui, Dang Gui* |
| **4. Tonify the qi to promote urination and invigorate the blood:**<br>• *Feng Shui* due to deficient and unstable protective qi with heavy sensation in the body, edema and dysuria. *+ Bai Zhu, Fang Ji*<br>• Sequelae of wind-stroke with qi deficiency and blood stasis manifested as hemiplegia. *+ Di Long, Dang Gui Wei* |
| **5. Used for Wasting and Thirsting Disorder and painful obstruction.** |

[Dosage] 10-15 g. 30-60 g. is permitted in special circumstances. Honey-fried to tonify and raise the yang; raw for all other conditions.

[Precautions] Not recommended in the cases of exterior excess, qi stagnation, damp obstruction, food stagnation, yin deficiency with heat signs, early stages of skin lesions, and skin conditions where heat toxins are present.

**Herbs that Tonify the Qi**

# Bai Zhu

*Rhizoma Atractylodis Macrocephalae*
*Bitter, sweet, warm; Spleen, Stomach*

*& Dⱥ'*

**[Characteristics]** It is sweet and warm to tonify qi of the middle burner, bitter to dry dampness, aromatic to strengthen the Spleen. It is often used to strengthen the Spleen and dry dampness in conditions of diarrhea, edema, and phlegm-dampness due to Spleen deficiency with dampness accumulation. It can also consolidate the surface to stop sweating and strengthen the Spleen to calm the fetus.

| FUNCTIONS • INDICATIONS & MAJOR COMBINATIONS |
|---|

**1. Tonify the Spleen and augment the qi:**
- Spleen and Stomach qi deficiency with fatigue, lack of appetite, abdominal distention and loose stool. *+ Ren Shen, Fu Ling*
- Middle burner deficient cold with abdominal pain, distention, diarrhea and vomiting. *+ Dang Shen, Gan Jiang*

**2. Strengthen the Spleen and dry dampness:**
- Spleen deficiency with loose stool or diarrhea. *+ Yi Yi Ren, Shan Yao*
- Spleen deficiency with congested fluids or edema. *+ Gui Zhi, Fu Ling*
- Spleen and Kidney yang deficiency with edema and reduced urination. *+ Fu Zi, Fu Ling*

**3. Consolidate the surface and stop sweating:**
- Qi deficiency with spontaneous sweating and recurrent colds. *+ Huang Qi, Fang Feng*

**4. Strengthen the Spleen and calm the fetus for Spleen deficiency with Restless Fetus Syndromes.**

**[Dosage]** 6-15 g. Raw to dry dampness and promote urination; dry-fried to tonify Spleen qi; scorched to strengthen the Spleen and stop diarrhea.

**[Comments]** ❶ Bai Zhu and Cang Zhu are both from the same family of Atractylodis, yet are different species. In ancient herbal documentation, Shen Nong Ben Cao Jing, there was only Zhu (Atracylodis) documented until Liang Dynasty.

❷ While Bai Zhu effectively strengthens the Spleen and tonifies the qi, dampness will be dried as a result. It also can stop sweating and calm the fetus. In contrary, Cang Zhu has a much stronger effect in drying dampness than strengthening the Spleen. It also induces sweating and releases the exterior. Consequently, in patterns of Spleen qi deficiency, Bai Zhu is more appropriate; whereas Cang Zhu is a much better choice for patterns of excessive dampness.

# Shan Yao

*Rhizoma Dioscoreae*
*Sweet, neutral; Spleen, Lung, Kidney*

[Characteristics] It evenly tonifies the qi and nourishes the yin of Lung, Spleen and Kidney. Additionally, it has the property of stabilizing and binding. Therefore, it is used to treat leakage of vital substances in various conditions of chronic cough due to Lung deficiency, loose stool due to Spleen deficiency, spermatorrhea and excessive vaginal discharge due to Kidney deficiency, as well as Wasting and Thirsting Disorder.

| FUNCTIONS • INDICATIONS & MAJOR COMBINATIONS |
|---|
| **1. Tonify the qi and nourish the yin:** <br> • Spleen qi deficiency with lack of appetite and loose watery stool. *+ Bai Zhu, Fu Ling* <br> • Lung and Kidney deficiency with chronic cough or wheezing. *+ Mai Men Dong, Wu Wei Zi* |
| **2. Tonify the Kidney and bind the essence:** <br> • Liver and Kidney yin deficiency with weakness of the lower extremities, night sweating and spermatorrhea. *+ Di Huang, Shan Zhu Yu* <br> • Kidney deficiency with frequent, copious urination and urinary incontinence. *+ Yi Zhi Ren, Wu Yao* <br> • Spleen deficiency and dampness accumulation or Kidney deficiency with excessive vaginal discharge. <br> — Cold-dampness. *+ Bai Zhu, Che Qian Zi* <br> — Damp-heat. *+ Huang Bai* |
| **3. Often used for Wasting and Thirsting Disorder, requiring large dose, decoct alone, or** *+ Tian Hua Fen, Ge Gen* |

[Dosage] 10-30 g, or up to 60-250 g. Raw to tonify the yin; dry-fried to strengthen the Spleen and stop diarrhea.

# Gan Cao

*Radix Glycyrrhizae*
*Sweet, neutral; Heart, Lung, Spleen, Stomach*

[Characteristics] Gan Cao is the representative of herbs with sweet property. Honey-fried form is sweet and warm to assist the yang, strengthen the Spleen and augment the Lung; raw form is cold to drain heat, reduce swelling and detoxify. By virtue of its sweet and moderating properties, it relaxes muscular spasms and alleviates pain, harmonizes and integrates the actions of other herbs in the prescription, and moderates the harsh properties of other herbs.

### FUNCTIONS • INDICATIONS & MAJOR COMBINATIONS

**1. Strengthen the Spleen and augment the qi:**
- Spleen and Stomach qi deficiency. *+ Ren Shen, Bai Zhu*
- Heart qi and blood deficiency with palpitation and irregular or intermittent pulse. *+ Gui Zhi, E Jiao*

**2. Moisten the Lung and stop coughing.**
- Wind-cold with cough. *+ Ma Huang, Xing Ren*
- Lung heat with cough. *+ Shi Gao, Ma Huang*
- Spleen deficiency generating phlegm with cough. *+ Ban Xia, Chen Pi*

**3. Clear heat and relieve fire toxicity:**
- Sore throat. *+ Jie Geng*
- Sores and carbuncles. *+ Jin Yin Hua, Pu Gong Ying*

**4. Moderate spasms and alleviate pain:**
- Spleen and Stomach deficient cold with spasmodic abdominal pain. *+ Yi Tang, Bai Shao*
- Blood deficiency or fluid consumption with cramps of the extremities. *+ Bai Shao*

[Dosage] 3-10 g. Raw to clear heat and detoxify; honey-fried for other purposes.

[Precautions] Contraindicated in excessive dampness. Long-term use may cause edema. Incompatible with Da Ji, Yuan Hua, Gan Sui and Hai Zao.

[Comments] ❶ It can also moderate the aggressive characteristics of other herbs; for instance, it can moderate the hot nature of Fu Zi, moderate the cold nature of Shi Gao, or moderate the purging nature of Da Huang.

❷ Most commonly used as an assistant or envoy in formulas for harmonizing and integrating the actions of other herbs. Due to its broad usage, it is known as "entering all twelve channels".

# Da Zao

*Fructus Jujubae*
*Sweet, warm; Spleen, Stomach*

[Characteristics] Its main functions are to strengthen the Spleen and Stomach, tonify the qi and blood. It also generates the fluid, harmonizes nutritive and protective qi, and moderates the aggressive characteristics of other herbs.

| FUNCTIONS • INDICATIONS & MAJOR COMBINATIONS |
|---|
| **1. Strengthen the Spleen and augment the qi:**<br>• Spleen and Stomach deficiency with shortness of breath, weakness, lack of appetite and loose stool. *+ Ren Shen, Bai Zhu* |
| **2. Nourish the blood and calm the spirit:**<br>• Blood deficiency with sallow complexion. *+ Shu Di Huang, Dang Gui*<br>• Restless Organ Disorder with irritability, frequent yawning, frequent episodes of melancholy and crying. *+ Gan Cao, Xiao Mai* |
| **3. Moderate the aggressive characteristics of other herbs.** |

[Dosage] 10-20 g.

[Precautions] This herb can retain dampness, generate heat and induce fullness of the middle burner. It is contraindicated in condition of epigastric and abdominal distention due to excessive dampness.

[Comments] ❶ The alternative name is Hong Zao.

❷ Da Zao is commonly combined with Sheng Jiang for mutual assistance. Da Zao can moderate the pungent and moving nature of Sheng Jiang, and Sheng Jiang can balance out the accumulative adverse effects of Da Zao. One tonifies while the other moves; one acts on the nutritive level while the other acts on the protective level. This combination supports the righteous qi, expels the pathogenic factors, and harmonizes the nutritive and protective qi.

# Huang Jing

*Rhizoma Polygonati*
*Sweet, neutral; Lung, Spleen, Kidney*

[Characteristics] It evenly tonifies the qi and yin of the Lung, Spleen and Kidney. It is often used for Spleen and Stomach deficiency, qi and yin deficiency.

**FUNCTIONS • INDICATIONS & MAJOR COMBINATIONS**

**1. Tonify Spleen qi and augment Stomach yin:**
- Spleen and Stomach qi deficiency with fatigue, general weakness and lack of appetite. *+ Dang Shen, Bai Zhu*
- Stomach yin deficiency with dry mouth, poor appetite and dry stools. *+ Sha Shen, Mai Men Dong*

**2. Moisten the Lung and nourish the yin:**
- Lung and Kidney yin deficiency with dry cough and scanty sputum. *+ Sha Shen, Bei Mu*

[Dosage] 10-30 g.

[Comments] In traditional textbooks, Huang Jing is categorized into yin tonics.

# Bai Bian Dou

*Semen Lablab Album*
*Sweet, slightly warm; Spleen, Stomach*

[Characteristics] It is often used to strengthen the Spleen and transform dampness. It also clears and relieves summerheat-dampness.

**FUNCTIONS • INDICATIONS & MAJOR COMBINATIONS**

**1. Strengthen the Spleen and transform dampness:**
- Spleen deficiency and excessive dampness with fatigue, chronic diarrhea and excessive vaginal discharge. *+ Ren Shen, Bai Zhu*

**2. Relieve summerheat and transform dampness:**
- Summerheat-dampness with vomiting and diarrhea. *+ Xiang Ru*

[Dosage] 10-20 g. Raw for summerheat; dry-fried for deficient Spleen qi with diarrhea.

[Comments] ❶ The alternative name is Bian Dou.
❷ Categorized into the herbs that clear heat in some textbooks.

# Feng Mi

*Mel*
*Sweet, neutral; Spleen, Lung, Large Intestine*

[Characteristics] Tonifies deficiency and moistens dryness. Characterized by its ability to moisten the Lung and strengthen the middle burner, it also lubricates the intestines and moderates spasmodic pain. Feng Mi is used to process other herbs to enhance their effects of tonifying and moistening. A common ingredient in pill form for formulas, Feng Mi can moderate the harsh effects of some herbs, as well as reduce the toxicity of other herbs.

| FUNCTIONS • INDICATIONS & MAJOR COMBINATIONS |
| --- |
| **1. Tonify the middle burner and moderate spasmodic pain:**<br>• Middle burner deficient cold with cold pain in the epigastrium and abdomen. *+ Bai Shao, Gui Zhi* |
| **2. Moisten the Lung and stop coughing:**<br>• Lung deficiency with chronic cough and dry throat. |
| **3. Lubricate the intestines to unblock the obstruction of bowel movements:**<br>• Intestinal dryness due to yin deficiency. *+ Dang Gui, Huo Ma Ren* |
| **4. Antidote for Wu Tou and Fu Zi.** |

[Dosage] 15-30 g. It can be dissolved in warm water or added to pills and syrup.

[Comments] The alternative name is Bai Mi.

# Yi Tang

*Saccharum Granorum*
*Sweet, warm; Lung, Spleen, Stomach*

[Characteristics] Sweet, warm and moist, it can tonify the deficiency and moderate spasmodic pain; it is often used for acute pain of the epigastric region and abdomen due to deficient cold, and dry cough due to Lung deficiency.

| FUNCTIONS • INDICATIONS & MAJOR COMBINATIONS |
| --- |
| **Tonify the qi, moderate spasm and alleviate pain:**<br>• Middle burner deficient cold with cold pain in the epigastrium and abdomen, eased with pressure or warmth. *+ Bai Shao, Gui Zhi* |

[Dosage] 30-60 g. Dissolved in the strained decoction.

# Shu Di Huang

*Radix Rehmanniae Preparata*
*Sweet, slightly warm; Liver, Kidney*

[Characteristics] Sweet, warm and cloying, it nourishes the yin and blood, as well as replenishes the essence and augments the marrow; therefore, it is the imperial herb for tonifying the Liver and Kidney, nourishing and securing the pre-heaven foundation. It is primarily used for conditions of the essence and blood deficiency.

**FUNCTIONS • INDICATIONS & MAJOR COMBINATIONS**

### 1. Tonify the blood and nourish the yin:

- Blood deficiency with sallow complexion, dizziness, insomnia, palpitation and irregular menstruation. *+ Dang Gui, Shao Yao*
- Kidney yin deficiency with tidal fever, five palms heat, night sweating, Wasting and Thirsting Disorder. *+ Shan Zhu Yu, Shan Yao*

### 2. Tonify the essence and augment the marrow:

- Kidney essence and blood deficiency with weakness of the lower back and knees, and premature graying. *+ He Shou Wu, Tu Si Zi*
- Kidney yin and essence insufficiency with weakness of the lower back and knees, dizziness and blurry vision. *+ Gou Qi Zi, Ju Hua*

[Dosage] 10-30 g.

[Comments] ❶ Add Sha Ren to counteract Shu Di Huang's cloying nature.

❷ Shu Di Huang, Xian Di Huang, and Sheng Di Huang are the same herbs processed in three various ways, therefore, having different effects. The following are the comparisons of these three herbs:

**Xian Di Huang**, with the bitter taste dominating the sweet taste, is also cold. Xian Di Huang has relatively stronger effects on clearing heat and cooling the blood. It is mostly used in conditions of thirst due to heat consuming the fluid, and for hemorrhages due to reckless movement of the blood.

**Sheng Di Huang**, with stronger sweet taste than bitter taste, has relatively greater effects on nourishing and moistening the yin than on clearing heat. It is mostly used in the conditions of yin deficiency with internal heat, and yin deficiency with internal dryness.

**Shu Di Huang**, slightly warm, is effective on tonifying the essence and blood, and is mainly used for essence and blood deficiency or consumptive deficiency. In conditions of essence and blood deficiency accompanied by yin deficiency with internal heat, Shu Di Huang is combined with Sheng Di Huang for mutual reinforcement, prescribed as Er Di, or two Di Huang.

# Dang Gui

*Radix Angelicae Sinensis*
*Sweet, acrid, warm; Liver, Heart, Spleen*

[Characteristics] It is the imperial herb for tonifying and invigorating the blood, and for regulating menses and alleviating pain. It is used in all patterns associated with blood deficiency, all types of pain associated with blood stasis, and irregular menstruation. It also nourishes the blood and moistens the intestines.

---

**FUNCTIONS • INDICATIONS & MAJOR COMBINATIONS**

### 1. Tonify and invigorate the blood:
- Patterns of blood deficiency. *+ Shu Di Huang, Bai Shao*
- Blood deficiency due to qi deficiency. *+ Huang Qi*
- Blood stasis with chest or abdominal pain. *+ Dan Shen, Chuan Xiong*
- Traumatic injuries with painul extremities. *+ Ru Xiang, Mo Yao*
- Wind-dampness Painful Obstruction. *+ Qiang Huo, Qin Jiao*

### 2. Regulate the menses and alleviate pain:
- Irregular menstruation, amenorrhea and dysmenorrhea.
  — Blood deficiency. *+ Shu Di'Huang, Bai Shao*
  — Blood stasis. *+ Tao Ren, Hong Hua*
  — Qi stagnation. *+ Xiang Fu, Yan Hu Suo*
  — Deficient cold. *+ Ai Ye, Gui Zhi*

### 3. Reduce swelling, expel pus and generate the tissue:
- Sores or abscesses. *+ Jin Yin Hua, Chi Shao*

### 4. Moisten the intestines, unblock the obstruction of bowel movements:
- Intestinal dryness due to blood deficiency with constipation.
  *+ Huo Ma Ren, He Shou Wu*

---

[Dosage] 6-12 g. Fry with wine to strengthen the effect in invigorating the blood.

[Precautions] Use with caution for abdominal distention and loose stool due to damp obstruction.

[Comments] ❶ To tonify the blood, use the body of Dang Gui; to invigorate the blood, use the tail of Dang Gui; to harmonize the blood (tonify and invigorate the blood), use the entire root of Dang Gui.

❷ There are two imperial herbs for regulating menses and alleviating pain— Dang Gui and Xiang Fu. Dang Gui tonifies and invigorates the blood and is used for irregular menstruation due to blood deficiency or blood stasis. Xiang Fu spreads Liver qi and is used for irregular menses due to constrained Liver qi.

# Bai Shao

*Radix Paeoniae Alba*
*Bitter, sour, slightly cold; Liver, Spleen*

[Characteristics] Sour and bitter, it enters the Liver channel. It nourishes Liver blood and preserves Liver yin, calms and curbs Liver yang and clears Liver fire, therefore a primary herb for all pathological patterns of the Liver, including deficiency of Liver yin and blood, and Liver yang rising.

**FUNCTIONS • INDICATIONS & MAJOR COMBINATIONS**

**1. Nourish the blood and preserve the yin:**
- Blood deficiency with sallow complexion, dizziness, palpitation or irregular menses. *+ Dang Gui, Shu Di Huang*
- Yin deficiency with night sweating. *+ Wu Wei Zi, Mu Li*
- Exterior deficiency, or disharmony between nutritive and protective qi with aversion to wind and sweating. *+ Gui Zhi*

**2. Soften and comfort the Liver and alleviate pain:**
- Blood deficiency and Liver qi stagnation with hypochondriac distention and pain. *+ Chai Hu, Dang Gui*
- Blood deficiency unable to nourish the sinews with spasmodic pain. *+ Gan Cao*
- Disharmony between the Liver and Spleen with recurrent abdominal pain and diarrhea. *+ Fang Feng, Bai Zhu*

**3. Calm and curb Liver yang:**
- Liver yin deficiency and Liver yang rising with irritability, short temper, headache and dizziness. *+ Shi Jue Ming, Niu Xi*

[Dosage] 6-15 g. May increase the dose to 15-30 g.

[Precautions] Incompatible with Li Lu.

[Comments] In ancient documentation and application, there were no distinctions between Bai Shao and Chi Shao. However, there is an obvious distinction between their individual functions and they are being used accordingly. The main function of Bai Shao is to nourish the blood and preserve the yin to soften the Liver, while the main functions of Chi Shao is to invigorate the blood and dispel blood stasis, clear heat and cool the blood. Both can alleviate pain; Bai Shao softens the Liver to stop pain while Chi Shao invigorates the blood and dispels stasis to alleviate pain.

# He Shou Wu

*Radix Polygoni Multiflori*
*Bitter, sweet, astringent, slightly warm; Liver, Kidney*

**[Characteristics]** Nourishes Liver blood, augments Kidney essence and binds the essence. Long-term usage of He Shou Wu is believed to prolong life. It is suitable for conditions known as "deficiency and unable to accept tonification". It is often used for essence and blood deficiency with premature graying or weakness in the lower back and knees. Fresh form can also detoxify, moisten the intestines and unblock the obstruction of bowel movements.

| FUNCTIONS • INDICATIONS & MAJOR COMBINATIONS |
| --- |

**1. Tonify the blood and essence:**
- Blood deficiency with sallow complexion, insomnia and forgetfulness. *+ Dang Gui, Suan Zao Ren*
- Deficiency of the essence and blood with weakness of the lower back and knees, blurry vision or premature graying. *+ Gou Qi Zi, Tu Si Zi*

**2. Relieve toxicity:**
- Heat accumulation with lumps around the neck such as goiter and scrofula. *+ Xia Ku Cao, Bei Mu*

**3. Moisten the intestines, unblock the obstruction of bowel movements:**
- Constipation due to blood deficiency and intestinal dryness. *+ Dang Gui, Huo Ma Ren*

**[Dosage]** 10-30 g. Fresh for stronger effects on relieving toxicity and moistening the intestines; honey-fried for tonifying the essence and blood.

**[Precautions]** Not recommended for loose stool and excessive phlegm-dampness.

**[Addendum]**
## Ye Jiao Teng
*Caulis Polygoni Multiflori*
The vine of the plant of He Shou Wu, also known as Shou Wu Teng, is sweet and neutral, and enters the Heart and Liver channels. It nourishes the Heart to calm the spirit and nourishes the blood to unblock the collaterals. It is used to treat insomnia due to yin and blood deficiency or soreness and pain of the extremities due to blood deficiency; the decoction is used as an external wash for skin rashes with itchiness. 15-30 g, increase the dose for topical application accordingly.

# E Jiao

*also enter chong & ren*

*Gelatinum Corii Asini*
*Sweet, neutral; Lung, Liver, Kidney*

**[Characteristics]** It nourishes Liver blood as well as augments Kidney yin. Due to its rich and cloying nature, it can promote coagulation to stop bleeding and is often used for bleeding caused by blood deficiency. It can also moisten the Lung.

**FUNCTIONS • INDICATIONS & MAJOR COMBINATIONS**

**1. Nourish the blood and stop bleeding:**
- Patterns of blood deficiency. *+ Dang Gui, Shu Di Huang*
- Hematemesis, epistaxis, blood in the stool, uterine bleeding, and various types of hemorrhaging.
  — Deficient cold. *+ Huang Qi, Ai Ye*
  — Heat in the blood. *+ Sheng Di Huang, Pu Huang*

**2. Nourish the yin and moisten dryness:**
- Dry cough due to Lung dryness and yin deficiency, and wheezing and coughing due to consumptive deficiency. *+ Sha Shen, Mai Dong*
- Yin injury with irritability and insomnia. *+ Huang Lian, Bai Shao*

**[Dosage]** 6-10 g. The strained decoction should be poured over the melted gelatin to dissolve it.

**[Precautions]** Not recommended for use in Spleen and Stomach deficiency.

**[Comments]** The alternative name is Lu Pi Jiao.

# Long Yan Rou

*Arillus Longan*
*Sweet, warm; Heart, Spleen*

**[Characteristics]** Augments the qi and blood, tonifies the Heart and Spleen, calms the spirit for insomnia due to deficiency of the Heart and Spleen.

**FUNCTIONS • INDICATIONS & MAJOR COMBINATIONS**

**Augment the qi and blood, tonify the Heart and Spleen:**
- Palpitation, anxiety, insomnia and forgetfulness due to Heart and Spleen deficiency. *+ Dang Shen, Dang Gui*

**[Dosage]** 10-15 g. May increase the dose to 30 g.

**[Comments]** The alternative name is Gui Yuan Rou.

# Gou Qi Zi

*Fructus Lycii*
*Sweet, neutral; Liver, Kidney, Lung*

[Characteristics] Evenly tonifies the Liver and Kidney, augments the essence and blood. It is primarily used for Liver and Kidney insufficiency, or deficiency of both the essence and blood. It also nourishes the Liver and enhances visual acuity.

| FUNCTIONS • INDICATIONS & MAJOR COMBINATIONS |
|---|
| **1. Nourish and tonify the Liver and Kidney:**<br>• Liver and Kidney deficiency with weakness of the lower back and knees, night sweating and nocturnal emission. *+ Di Huang, Tu Si Zi* |
| **2. Nourish the Liver and enhance visual acuity:**<br>• Liver and Kidney yin deficiency with dry eyes, blurry vision and decreased visual acuity. *+ Di Huang, Ju Hua* |
| **3. Moisten the Lung:**<br>• Yin deficiency with chronic cough. *+ Mai Men Dong, Zhi Mu* |

[Dosage] 6-10 g.


# Sang Shen

*Fructus Mori*
*Sweet, cold; Heart, Liver, Kidney*

[Characteristics] Nourishes the yin and tonifies the blood; this tonic herb is not cloying. It is used in the patterns of yin and blood deficiency. It also generates the fluid, moistens the intestines and unblocks the obstruction of bowel movements.

| FUNCTIONS • INDICATIONS & MAJOR COMBINATIONS |
|---|
| **1. Nourish the yin and tonify the blood:**<br>• Yin and blood deficiency with premature graying. Use alone (decoct first then add Feng Mi and simmer to syrup). |
| **2. Generate the fluid and moisten the intestines:**<br>• Wasting and Thirsting Disorder. *+ Mai Men Dong, Tian Hua Fen*<br>• Yin and blood deficiency with constipation. *+ Huo Ma Ren* |

[Dosage] 10-15 g. Up to 15-30 g. when using syrup form. Pour warm water over the syrup in the container; stir well prior to administration.

# Sha Shen

*Radix Glehniae seu Adenophorae*
*Sweet, slightly bitter, slightly cold; Lung, Stomach*

[Characteristics] Mainly enters the Lung and Stomach channels; it clears heat and nourishes the yin. It is often used for dry cough caused by Lung dryness and yin deficiency, dry throat and thirst caused by Stomach dryness and Warm-Febrile Disease injuring the yin.

**FUNCTIONS • INDICATIONS & MAJOR COMBINATIONS**

### 1. Clear Lung heat and moisten Lung yin:
- Heat injuring Lung yin with dry cough and thirst. *+ Mai Men Dong, Yu Zhu*
- Lung yin deficiency with dry cough, blood-tinged sputum and hoarseness. *+ Zhi Mu, Bei Mu*

### 2. Nourish the Stomach and generate the fluid:
- Yin injured by Warm-Febrile Disease with thirst, dry throat, poor appetite and dry stool. *+ Mai Men Dong, Sheng Di Huang*
- Severe cases of Warm-Febrile Disease injuring the yin with thirst, dry throat and dark red tongue. Use Xian Sha Shen *+ Xian Di Huang*

[Dosage] 10-15 g. May increase the dose to 15-30 g when using fresh form.

[Precautions] Incompatible with Li Lu.

[Comments] There are two species of Sha Shen— Nan Sha Shen and Bei Sha Shen. Both clear heat and nourish the yin of the Lung and Stomach. The fresh form of Nan Sha Shen is called Xian Sha Shen. Differentiations among these three are:

**Bei Sha Shen** has relatively stronger effects in nourishing the yin and moistening the Lung.

**Nan Sha Shen** has relatively greater effects on clearing the Lung and dispelling phlegm.

**Xian Sha Shen** is more effective on clearing heat and generating the fluid. Therefore, it is often used in treating thirst due to heat injuring yin.

# Mai Men Dong

*Radix Ophiopogonis*
*Sweet, slightly bitter, slightly cold; Heart, Lung, Stomach*

[Characteristics] It nourishes the yin, clears heat, generates the fluid and moistens dryness. It moistens the Lung and nourishes Stomach yin. It also enters the Heart channel to clear heat and eliminate irritability. It is often used for dry cough caused by Lung dryness, thirst caused by yin injury, and irritability caused by yin deficiency with heat.

| FUNCTIONS • INDICATIONS & MAJOR COMBINATIONS |
| --- |

**1. Nourish the yin and moisten the Lung:**
- Dry-heat injuring the Lung with dry throat and nose, and sticky sputum. *+ Sang Ye, Xing Ren*
- Lung and Kidney yin deficiency causing heat with dry cough, sticky and blood-tinged sputum. *+ Tian Men Dong*

**2. Nourish the Stomach and generate the fluid:**
- Stomach yin deficiency with thirst, dry tongue and mouth. *+ Sha Shen, Yu Zhu*
- Yin deficiency and dryness of the intestines with constipation. *+ Sheng Di Huang, Xuan Shen*

**3. Clear the Heart and eliminate irritability:**
- Yin deficiency causing heat with irritability and insomnia. *+ Sheng Di Huang, Suan Zao Ren*
- Nutritive level of Warm-Febrile Disease with fever worse at night, irritability and restlessness. *+ Sheng Di Huang, Huang Lian*

[Dosage] 10-15 g.

[Comments] ❶ The alternative names are Mai Dong and Cun Dong.

❷ Used with the core of the herb for clearing heat from the Heart and eliminating irritability; used without the core for clearing heat and nourishing yin of the Lung and Stomach.

# Tian Men Dong

*Radix Asparagi*
*Sweet, bitter, very cold; Lung, Kidney*

**[Characteristics]** Mainly enters the Lung and Kidney channels; it is extremely cold. It has strong effects to clear heat, nourish the yin and moisten dryness.

| FUNCTIONS • INDICATIONS & MAJOR COMBINATIONS |
| --- |

**1. Clear Lung heat and drain fire:**
- Dry cough with sticky sputum or consumptive cough with hemoptysis. *+ Mai Men Dong*

**2. Nourish the yin and moisten dryness:**
- Heat injuring the yin with thirst or fluid consumption with Wasting and Thirsting Disorder. *+ Ren Shen, Sheng Di Huang*

**[Dosage]** 6-15 g.

**[Precautions]** Contraindicated in Spleen and Stomach deficient cold.

**[Comments]** The alternative name is Tian Dong.

# Yu Zhu

*Rhizoma Polygonati Odorati*
*Sweet, slightly cold; Lung, Stomach*

**[Characteristics]** With similar effects as Sha Shen in generating the fluid and moistening dryness, this yin tonic herb does not retain pathogenic factors; therefore, it is used to treat exterior wind-heat in pre-existing yin deficiency.

| FUNCTIONS • INDICATIONS & MAJOR COMBINATIONS |
| --- |

**1. Nourish the yin and moisten the Lung:**
- Lung dryness with dry cough. *+ Sha Shen, Mai Men Dong*
- Exterior wind-heat in pre-existing yin deficiency with headache and severe thirst. *+ Bo He, Dan Dou Chi*

**2. Generate the fluid and alleviate thirst:**
- Warm-Febrile Disease injuring the fluid with irritability, thirst, dry mouth and tongue. *+ Sha Shen, Mai Men Dong*

**[Dosage]** 10-15 g.

**[Comments]** The alternative name is Wei Rui.

# Shi Hu

*Herba Dendrobii*
*Sweet, slightly cold; Stomach, Kidney*

**[Characteristics]** Characterized by its ability to nourish Stomach yin and clear deficient heat, it is used in Warm-Febrile Disease injuring the yin and yin deficiency with persistent fever. It is also used to enhance visual acuity.

| FUNCTIONS • INDICATIONS & MAJOR COMBINATIONS |
|---|
| **1. Nourish Stomach yin and generate the fluid:**<br>• Warm-Febrile Disease injuring the yin or Stomach yin deficiency with dry mouth and thirst. *+ Sheng Di Huang, Mai Men Dong* |
| **2. Nourish the yin and clear heat:**<br>• Yin deficiency and fluid consumption with chronic persistent fever. *+ Sheng Di Huang, Bai Wei* |
| **3. Enhance visual acuity.** *+ Ju Hua, Gou Qi Zi* |

**[Dosage]** 6-15 g. Up to 15-30 g when using fresh form. Decoct first.

**[Precautions]** Contraindicated in early stage of Warm-Febrile Disease and unresolved damp-heat because this herb retains pathogenic factors, especially dampness.


# Bai He

*Bulbus Lilii*
*Sweet, slightly cold; Lung, Heart*

**[Characteristics]** It moistens the Lung and clears heat from the Heart. It is often used for dry cough due to Lung dryness, and also for irritability and insomnia.

| FUNCTIONS • INDICATIONS & MAJOR COMBINATIONS |
|---|
| **1. Moisten the Lung and stop coughing:**<br>• Lung yin deficiency with heat manifesting with dry cough and blood-tinged sputum. *+ Sheng Di Huang, Xuan Shen* |
| **2. Clear heat from the Heart and calm the spirit:**<br>• Late stage of Warm-Febrile Disease accompanied with residual heat manifesting with irritability and insomnia. *+ Sheng Di Huang* |

**[Dosage]** 10-30 g.

*Han Lian Cao*

# Mo Han Lian

*Herba Ecliptae*
*Sweet, sour, cold; Liver, Kidney*

**[Characteristics]** Tonifies Liver and Kidney yin as well as cools the blood and stops bleeding. It is often used in the cases of Liver and Kidney yin deficiency, yin deficiency with heat signs, and bleeding due to heat in the blood.

**FUNCTIONS • INDICATIONS & MAJOR COMBINATIONS**

**1. Nourish and tonify the Liver and Kidney:**
- Liver and Kidney yin deficiency with dizziness, tinnitus and premature graying. *+ Nu Zhen Zi*

**2. Cool the blood and stop bleeding:**
- Yin deficiency accompanied with heat in the blood with subcutaneous and mucosa bleeding, blood in the stool, hematuria, and Gushing and Leaking Syndromes. *+ Sheng Di Huang, Bai Mao Gen*
- For traumatic injuries with bleeding, smash the fresh herb and apply it topically.

**[Dosage]** 10-15 g. Double the dose when using fresh form.
**[Comments]** The alternative name is Han Lian Cao.


# Nu Zhen Zi

*Fructus Ligustri Lucidi*
*Sweet, bitter, cool; Liver, Kidney*

**[Characteristics]** Mildly tonifies Liver and Kidney yin; it treats patterns of Liver and Kidney yin deficiency. Due to its mild nature, it can be taken long-term.

**FUNCTIONS • INDICATIONS & MAJOR COMBINATIONS**

**1. Nourish and tonify the Liver and Kidney:**
- Liver and Kidney yin deficiency with dizziness, tinnitus and premature graying. *+ Han Lian Cao*

**2. Nourish the Liver and enhance visual acuity:**
- Liver yin insufficiency with decreased visual acuity and blurry vision. *+ Ju Hua, Gou Qi Zi*

**[Dosage]** 10-15 g.

# Gui Ban

*Carapax et Plastrum Testudinis*
*Salty, sweet, cold; Liver, Kidney, Heart* ✝ *R ● ⌐*

[Characteristics] Gui Ban is an animal product that is used as an herb with direct tonifying effects on vital substances. It acts on the Conception channel and greatly tonifies Kidney yin and anchors the yang, as well as benefits the Kidney and strengthens the bones. Gui Ban is often used in the patterns of Kidney yin deficiency, Steaming Bone Disorder, internal movement of deficient wind, Liver yang rising, and weakness of the bones due to Kidney deficiency.

| FUNCTIONS ● INDICATIONS & MAJOR COMBINATIONS |
| --- |
| **1. Nourish the yin and anchor the yang:** <br>• Yin deficiency accompanied by empty fire with Steaming Bone Disorder and night sweating. *+ Shu Di Huang, Zhi Mu* <br>• Yin deficiency of the Liver and Kidney accompanied by ascending yang with dizziness and vertigo. *+ Sheng Di Huang, Shi Jue Ming* <br>• Yin deficiency accompanied by internal movement of wind with dizziness, vertigo and irritability. *+ E Jiao, Sheng Di Huang* |
| **2. Benefit the Kidney and strengthen the bones:** <br>• Soreness of the lower back, weakness of the lower extremities, and delayed skeletal development in children. *+ Niu Xi, Suo Yang* |
| **3. Treat bleeding and prevent excessive menstruation for yin deficiency causing heat with Gushing and Leaking Syndromes.** |

[Dosage] 10-30 g. Decoct first.

[Precautions] Contraindicated in Spleen deficient cold and during pregnancy.

[Comments] Clinically, Gui Ban is often combined with Lu Rong. For differentiation and application (p. 230).

[Addendum]
## Gui Ban Jiao
*Gelatinum Carapax et Plastrum Testudinis*
The gelatin form of Gui Ban is made by simmering Gui Ban for an extensive period of time. It has the same property and similar effects as Gui Ban, but it is richer and more cloying. It has greater effects on nourishing Kidney yin and stopping hemorrhages; therefore, it is specifically appropriate for soreness and weakness of the lower back and bleeding due to Kidney deficiency. It is often combined with Lu Jiao Jiao. For differentiation and application (p. 231).

# Bie Jia

*Carapax Trionycis*
*Salty, cold; Liver*

[Characteristics] Salty and cold, it enters the Kidney channel. Bie Jia nourishes the yin, anchors the yang and clears heat. It is relatively weaker in nourishing the yin yet stronger in clearing heat compared to Gui Ban. It also enters the blood level of the Liver and Spleen to invigorate the blood, soften hardness and dissipate nodules.

| FUNCTIONS • INDICATIONS & MAJOR COMBINATIONS |
| --- |

**1. Nourish the yin and anchor the yang:**
- Warm-Febrile Disease injuring the yin accompanied by internal movement of deficient wind. *+ Mu Li, E Jiao*
- Late stage of Warm-Febrile Disease, heat lingering in the nutritive and blood level, with fever at night and absence of sweating as fever reduces. *+ Qing Hao, Sheng Di Huang*
- Yin deficiency with Steaming Bone Disorder. *+ Di Gu Pi, Zhi Mu*

**2. Soften hardness and dissipate nodules:**
- Amenorrhea and *Zheng Jia*. *+ Da Huang, Hu Po*
- Chronic malarial disorder with hepatosplenomegaly. *+ Chai Hu, Zhe Chong*

[Dosage] 10-30 g. Decoct first; raw to nourish the yin and anchor the yang; vinegar-fried to soften hardness and dissipate nodules.

[Precautions] Contraindicated in Spleen and Stomach deficient cold and during pregnancy.

# Lu Rong

*Cornu Cervi Pantotrichum*
*Sweet, salty, warm; Liver, Kidney* + Du

[Characteristics] Tonifies the Governing vessel, stabilizes the Penetrating and Conception vessels. Lu Rong is the ultimate tonic herb for the Liver and Kidney. Characterized by its abilities to fortify Kidney yang, augment the essence and blood, and strengthen the sinews and bones, it is primarily used for Kidney yang insufficiency, essence and blood deficiency, weakness of the sinews and bones, developmental delayed in children, Gushing and Leaking Syndromes and excessive vaginal discharge due to unstable Penetrating and Conception vessels. Moreover, it generates the tissue and promotes healing process to treat yin-type of abscesses.

| FUNCTIONS • INDICATIONS & MAJOR COMBINATIONS |
|---|
| **1. Tonify the Kidney and fortify the yang:** <br> • Kidney yang insufficiency with cold pain at the lower back and knees, frequent urination, impotence and premature ejaculation or infertility due to cold womb. May use alone in powdered form, or take the pill form. *+ Ren Shen, Shu Di Huang* |
| **2. Augment the essence and blood, and strengthen the sinews and bones:** <br> • Essence and blood deficiency with lack of strength of the sinews and bones or physical and mental developmental delayed in children. *+ Shu Di Huang, Shan Yao* |
| **3. Stabilize the Penetrating and Conception vessels:** <br> • Deficient cold of the Penetrating and Conception vessels with unremitting Gushing and Leaking Syndromes. *+ E Jiao, Pu Huang* <br> • Unstable Girdle vessel with deficient cold type of excessive vaginal discharge. *+ Gou Ji, Bai Lian* |
| **4. Non-healing ulcerations and sores or non-perforated yin-type of abscesses due to qi and blood deficiency.** |

[Dosage] 1-3 g. Use the powdered or pill forms. Initiate with low dose and gradually increase the dose.

[Precautions] Contraindicated in yin deficiency with heat signs.

[Comments] Both Lu Rong and Gui Ban tonify the Kidney and strengthen the sinews and bones. Gui Ban nourishes Kidney yin and acts on the Conception vessel; it can nourish the yin and anchor the yang, tonify the blood and stop bleeding. It is appropriate for patterns of heat in the blood with Gushing and Leaking Syndromes, and yin deficiency with heat. Lu Rong, on the other hand, fortifies

230

Kidney yang and tonifies the Governing vessel; it can warm the Kidney, fortify the yang, generate the essence and benefit the marrow. It is suitable for patterns of deficient cold with Gushing and Leaking Syndromes, and yang deficiency with fear of cold. In the case of deficiency of both yin and yang, use both Gui Ban and Lu Rong together.

## [Addendum]
## Lu Jiao
### *Cornu Cervi*
Ossified horn of Cervus nippon Temminck or C. elaphus L., Lu Jiao is salty and warm, and it enters the Liver and Kidney channels. It tonifies the Kidney, fortifies the yang and substitutes for Lu Rong with relatively weaker effects. It also invigorates the blood and reduces swelling; therefore, it is used for toxic swelling and sores, breast abscess, and pain due to blood stasis. 6-10 g. Contraindicated in yin deficiency with heat.

## Lu Jiao Jiao
### *Gelatinum Cornu Cervi*
Lu Jiao Jiao is the gelatin form of Lu Jiao made by simmering until it concentrates. It is sweet, salty and warm, and it enters the Liver and Kidney channels. It tonifies Kidney yang, augments the essence and blood, and effectively stops bleeding; therefore, it is used for essence and blood deficiency, and deficient cold with bleeding. 6-10 g. Pour the strained decoction over the melted gelatin to dissolve it. Contraindicated in yin deficiency with heat.

Both Lu Jiao Jiao and Gui Ban Jiao are herbs made from animal derivatives that have direct effects on the vital substances. Lu Jiao Jiao tonifies the yang while Gui Ban Jiao nourishes the yin. Known as "Gui Lu Er Xian Jiao", they replenish the Conception and Governing vessels, and greatly tonify the essence and blood when these two herbs are combined.

## Lu Jiao Shuang
### *Cornu Cervi Degelatinatum*
The residue of Lu Jiao after simmering, with relatively weaker function on tonifying Kidney yang and stronger binding effects, it is used to stop uterine bleeding and excessive vaginal discharge. When it is applied topically, it treats chronic non-healing sores. 10-15 g. Contraindicated in yin deficiency with heat.

# Ba Ji Tian

*Radix Morindae Officinalis*
*Acrid, sweet, warm; Kidney, Liver*

[Characteristics] Tonifies Kidney yang, augments the essence, and strongly strengthens the sinews and bones; it treats lower burner deficient cold with weakness of the sinews and bones. It also disperses cold-dampness.

| FUNCTIONS • INDICATIONS & MAJOR COMBINATIONS |
|---|
| **1. Tonify the Kidney and fortify the yang:** <br> • Insufficient Kidney yang with cold pain in the lower abdomen, impotence or cold womb infertility. *+ Xian Mao, Yin Yang Huo* |
| **2. Strengthen the sinews and bones, and disperse cold-dampness:** <br> • Wind-cold-damp Painful Obstruction with pain and weakness of the lower back and lower extremities. *+ Du Zhong, Sang Ji Sheng* |

[Dosage] 6-15 g.

[Precautions] Contraindicated in yin deficiency with heat.


# Yin Yang Huo

*Herba Epimedii*
*Acrid, sweet, warm; Liver, Kidney*

[Characteristics] It tonifies Kidney yang to strengthen the sinews and bones; it also strongly disperses cold-damp to unblock painful obstruction. It is often used in patterns of Kidney yang deficiency and Wind-cold-damp Painful Obstruction.

| FUNCTIONS • INDICATIONS & MAJOR COMBINATIONS |
|---|
| **1. Tonify the Kidney and fortify the yang:** <br> • Insufficient Kidney yang with cold pain in the lower abdomen, impotence or cold womb infertility. *+ Xian Mao, Ba Ji Tian* |
| **2. Disperse cold and dispel dampness:** <br> • Wind-cold-damp Painful Obstruction with pain and weakness of the lower back and lower extremities. *+ Ba Ji Tian, Du Zhong* |

[Dosage] 6-10 g.

[Precautions] Contraindicated in yin deficiency with heat.

[Comments] The alternative name is Xian Ling Pi.

# Xian Mao

*Rhizoma Curculiginis*
*Acrid, hot, toxic; Kidney*

[Characterisitcs] An acrid, hot and toxic herb with aggressive actions, it is an important herb for tonifying the Kidney and fortifying the yang. It is primarily used for the failure of fire in the Gate of Vitality. It also disperses cold-damp.

**FUNCTIONS • INDICATIONS & MAJOR COMBINATIONS**

### 1. Tonify the Kidney and fortify the yang:
- Insufficient Kidney yang with impotence, premature ejaculation and male infertility. *+ Yin Yang Huo, Lu Rong*

### 2. Used in Wind-cold-damp Painful Obstruction.

[Dosage] 3-10 g.

[Precautions] Do not exceed the recommended dose; not for long-term use.

# Rou Cong Rong

*Herba Cistanches*
*Sweet, salty, warm; Kidney, Large Intestine*

[Characteristics] Sweet, warm and moist, it warms Kidney yang and augments Kidney essence. It can be used in the patterns of Kidney yang insufficiency, essence and blood deficiency. It also moistens dryness in the intestines.

**FUNCTIONS • INDICATIONS & MAJOR COMBINATIONS**

### 1. Tonify the Kidney and assist the yang:
- Insufficient Kidney yang and deficiency of the essence and blood.
  — Impotence and premature ejaculation. *+ Tu Si Zi, Wu Wei Zi*
  — Cold womb and female infertility. *+ Lu Jiao Jiao, Zi He Chè*
  — Soreness and weakness of the lower back and lower extremities. *+ Ba Ji Tian, Du Zhong*

### 2. Moisten the intestines and unblock the obstruction of bowel movements:
- Yang deficiency, insufficiency of the essence and blood, and dryness of the intestines with constipation. *+ Dang Gui, Sheng Ma*

[Dosage] 10-20 g. Large dose is permitted because of its moderate effects.

[Precautions] Contraindicated in yin deficiency with heat and loose stool.

# Suo Yang

*Herba Cynomorii*
*Sweet, warm; Liver, Kidney, Large Intestine*

[Characteristics] Sweet, warm and moist, it has similar effects as Rou Cong Rong. It strongly nourishes the sinews to improve the conditions of motor impairment and muscular atrophy. It also moistens the intestines.

FUNCTIONS • INDICATIONS & MAJOR COMBINATIONS

**1. Tonify the Kidney and assist the yang:**
   • Kidney yang and essence deficiency with soreness and weakness of the sinews and bones. + *Shu Di Huang, Gui Ban*

**2. For intestinal dryness with constipation, use this herb alone (decoct first, add Feng Mi and simmer to syrup).**

[Dosage] 10-15 g

[Precautions] Contraindicated in yin deficiency with heat signs, diarrhea due to Spleen deficiency, and constipation due to excess heat.


# Du Zhong

*Cortex Eucommiae*
*Sweet, warm; Liver, Kidney*

[Characteristics] Tonifies the Liver and Kidney, strengthens the sinews and bones; it also augments the Liver and Kidney to calm the fetus.

FUNCTIONS • INDICATIONS & MAJOR COMBINATIONS

**1. Tonify the Liver and Kidney, and strengthen the sinews and bones:**
   • Insufficiency of the Liver and Kidney with weak, sore or painful lower back and knees. + *Xu Duan, Niu Xi*
   • Liver and Kidney deficient cold with impotence and frequent urination. + *Bu Gu Zhi, Tu Si Zi*

**2. Calm the fetus:**
   • Liver and Kidney insufficiency or deficient Penetrating and Conception vessels with Restless Fetus Syndromes. + *E Jiao, Xu Duan*

[Dosage] 10-15 g. Fry with salt-water to enhance the effect of tonifying Kidney.

[Precautions] Use with caution in heat conditions from yin deficiency.

**Herbs that Tonify the Yang**

# Xu Duan

*Radix Dipsaci*
*Bitter, sweet, acrid, slightly warm; Liver, Kidney*

[Characteristics] Tonifies the Liver and Kidney, promotes the movement of blood and mends the sinews and bones to treat fracture. It also calms the fetus. Xu Duan is an important herb for obstetric/gynecologic and orthopedic disorders. It is used for soreness and weakness of the lower back and knees, injuries of the sinews and bones, Gushing and Leaking Syndromes, and Restless Fetus Syndromes.

| FUNCTIONS • INDICATIONS & MAJOR COMBINATIONS |
|---|
| **1. Tonify the Liver and Kidney:** <br>• Deficiency of the Liver and Kidney with sore and painful lower back and knees. *+ Du Zhong, Niu Xi* <br>• Wind-cold-damp Painful Obstruction with painful joints, sore and weak lower back and knees. *+ Fang Feng, Niu Xi* |
| **2. Promote the movement of blood, and the mending of sinews and bones:** <br>• Fracture due to traumatic injuries. *+ Gu Sui Bu, Xue Jie* |
| **3. Calm the fetus and stop spotting:** <br>• Pregnant woman with significant lower back pain and spotting or habitual miscarriage. *+ Sang Ji Sheng, Tu Si Zi* |

[Dosage] 10-20 g. Fried form for uterine bleeding; powder for topical application.

[Comments] ❶ The alternative name is Chuan Xu Duan.

❷ Xu Duan is an effective herb to calm the fetus. Restless Fetus Syndromes can result from various pathogenesis; therefore, herbs that calms the fetus have different indications. Common herbs that calm the fetus are:

**Zi Su** and **Sha Ren** facilitates the movements of qi and calms the fetus; they are used for Restless Fetus Syndromes due to qi stagnation.

**Huang Qin** clears heat to calm the fetus; it is used for Restless Fetus Syndromes due to warm womb.

**Ai Ye** warms the meridians and stops bleeding to calm the fetus; it is used for Restless Fetus Syndromes due to cold womb.

**Bai Zhu** strengthens the Spleen to calm the fetus; it is used for Restless Fetus Syndromes due to Spleen deficiency.

**Sang Ji Sheng**, **Du Zhong**, **Xu Duan** and **Tu Si Zi** all tonify the Liver and Kidney to calm the fetus; they are used for Restless Fetus Syndromes due to unstable Penetrating and Conception vessels.

# Gu Sui Bu

*Rhizoma Drynariae*
*Bitter, warm; Liver, Kidney*

[Characteristics] In addition to its ability of tonifying the Kidney, it can effectively promote the movement of blood to treat traumatic injuries. It can be taken internally or applied externally.

| FUNCTIONS • INDICATIONS & MAJOR COMBINATIONS |
|---|
| **1. Tonify the Kidney:** |
| • Patterns of Kidney deficiency. |
| — Soreness and weakness of the lower back and knees. *+ Bu Gu Zhi* |
| — Tinnitus or deafness. *+ Shu Di Huang, Shan Zhu Yu* |
| **2. Promote the movement of blood and the mending of sinews and bones:** |
| • Fracture, strain and/or sprain of muscles and tendons due to traumatic injuries. *+ Zi Ran Tong, Mo Yao* |

[Dosage] 10-20 g. Apply the tincture topically for alopecia.

[Precautions] Not recommended for yin deficiency with heat signs or those without blood stasis.

# Gou Ji

*Rhizoma Cibotii*
*Bitter, sweet, warm; Liver, Kidney*

[Characteristics] Tonifies the Liver and Kidney, strengthens the lower back and spine. It also can expel wind-cold-damp for painful obstruction.

| FUNCTIONS • INDICATIONS & MAJOR COMBINATIONS |
|---|
| **1. Tonify the Liver and Kidney, strengthen the lower back and spine:** |
| • Deficient Liver and Kidney accompanied by Wind-cold-damp Painful Obstruction with lower back pain, stiffness of the spine and weakness of the lower extremities. *+ Du Zhong, Xu Duan* |
| **2. Urinary incontinence or excessive vaginal discharge.** |

[Dosage] 10-15 g.

[Precautions] Contraindicated in conditions of internal heat.

[Comments] The fur of Gou Ji stops bleeding and generates the tissue.

# Bu Gu Zhi

*Fructus Psoraleae*
*Acrid, bitter, very warm; Kidney, Spleen*

[Characteristics] Acrid, bitter and very warm in nature, it also has an astringent property. It is an important herb for Spleen and Kidney yang deficiency, the failure of fire in the Gate of Vitality, and unstable lower burner; it also assists the Kidney to grasp the qi for cold type wheezing and coughing.

| FUNCTIONS • INDICATIONS & MAJOR COMBINATIONS |
|---|
| **1. Tonify the Kidney and assist the yang:** |
| • Kidney yang deficiency with cold and pain or soreness and weakness of the lower back and knees. *+ Du Zhong, Hu Tao Rou* |
| • Kidney yang deficiency with impotence. *+ Tu Si Zi, Hu Tao Rou* |
| **2. Secure the essence and restrain the leakage:** |
| • Spermatorrhea, frequent urination and enuresis. *+ Xiao Hui Xiang* |
| **3. Warm the Spleen and stop diarrhea:** |
| • Spleen and Kidney yang deficiency with daybreak diarrhea. *+ Rou Dou Kou, Wu Wei Zi* |
| **4. Kidney deficiency unable to grasp the qi with wheezing.** *+ Hu Tao Rou* |

[Dosage] 6-10 g.

[Precautions] Contraindicated in yin deficiency with heat or constipation.

[Comments] The alternative name is Po Gu Zhi.

# Tu Si Zi

*Semen Cuscutae*
*Acrid, sweet, neutral; Liver, Kidney*

[Characteristics] Tu Si Zi evenly tonifies Kidney yin as well as Kidney yang; it also binds the essence. In addition, it augments the Liver to improve vision, warms the Spleen to stop diarrhea, and stabilizes the Penetrating and Conception vessels to calm the fetus.

| FUNCTIONS • INDICATIONS & MAJOR COMBINATIONS |
|---|
| **1. Tonify the yang, augment the yin, secure the essence and restrain leakage:**<br>• Kidney deficiency and unstable lower burner.<br>— Impotence and nocturnal emission. *+ Gou Qi Zi, Wu Wei Zi*<br>— Urinary incontinence. *+ Lu Rong, Sang Piao Xiao*<br>— Cloudy urine and excessive vaginal discharge. *+ Lian Zi, Qian Shi* |
| **2. Nourish the Liver and enhance visual acuity:**<br>• Insufficiency of the Liver and Kidney with blurry vision. *+ Shu Di Huang, Che Qian Zi* |
| **3. Warm the Spleen and stop diarrhea:**<br>• Spleen deficiency with diarrhea or loose stool. *+ Huang Qi, Dang Shen* |
| **4. Calm the fetus:**<br>• Liver and Kidney insufficiency with habitual or threatened miscarriage. *+ Xu Duan, Sang Ji Sheng* |

[Dosage] 10-15 g.

[Precautions] Not recommended for use in yin deficiency with heat signs, constipation, and dark scanty urine.

# Yi Zhi Ren

*Fructus Alpiniae Oxyphyllae*
*Acrid, warm; Spleen, Kidney*

[Characteristics] It warms and tonifies, as well as stabilizes and binds. It warms the Spleen and Stomach, harmonizes the middle burner, and limits excessive salivation. It also warms Kidney yang and stabilizes the lower burner.

**FUNCTIONS • INDICATIONS & MAJOR COMBINATIONS**

**1. Warm the Spleen and Stomach, and stop drooling:**
   - Spleen and Stomach deficient cold with poor appetite, diarrhea, excessive salivation and drooling. *+ Dang Shen, Bai Zhu*

**2. Tonify Kidney yang and secure the essence:**
   - Kidney yang deficiency with spermatorrhea, enuresis, frequent copious urination and dribbling of urine. *+ Shan Yao, Wu Yao*

[Dosage] 3-10 g.

[Precautions] Contraindicated in yin deficiency with heat.


# Sha Yuan Zi

*Semen Astragali Complanati*
*Sweet, warm; Liver, Kidney*

[Characteristics] Mildly tonifies the Liver and Kidney and it has an astringent property. It also improves visual acuity.

**FUNCTIONS • INDICATIONS & MAJOR COMBINATIONS**

**1. Tonify the Kidney and secure the essence:**
   - Kidney deficiency with sore and weak lower extremities, spermatorrhea and excessive vaginal discharge. *+ Long Gu, Qian Shi*

**2. Nourish the Liver and enhance visual acuity:**
   - Insufficiency of the Liver and Kidney with dizziness and blurry vision. *+ Gou Qi Zi, Ju Hua*

[Dosage] 10-20 g.

[Precautions] Contraindicated in yin deficiency with heat signs, and in urinary difficulties.

[Comments] The alternative name is Sha Yuan Ji Li.

# Zi He Che

*Placenta Hominis*
*Sweet, salty, warm; Lung, Liver, Kidney*

[Characteristics] It is a good tonic for the yin, yang, qi and blood. Combined with the appropriate herbs, Zi He Che can treat all patterns of deficiency. Because of its mild effects, it is more beneficial to be taken long-term.

| FUNCTIONS • INDICATIONS & MAJOR COMBINATIONS |
|---|
| **1. Tonify the essence:**<br>• Patterns of Kidney insufficiency or essence and blood deficiency with impotence, nocturnal emission, dizziness, tinnitus, soreness and weakness of the lower back and knees. Often combined with other tonics. |
| **2. Nourish the blood and augment the qi:**<br>• Qi and blood deficiency with emaciation and sallow complexion. *+ Dang Gui, Huang Qi* |
| **3. Augment the Lung and Kidney, and promote the grasp of qi:**<br>• Lung and Kidney deficiency and Kidney unable to grasp the qi with wheezing and coughing. *+ Ren Shen, Ge Jie* |

[Dosage] 1.5-3 g. Take the powdered form with warm water; or add in pills.

[Comments] The alternative name is Tai Pan.

## [Remarks & Differentiations]

### Ren Shen — Dang Shen

| | Ren Shen | Dang Shen |
|---|---|---|
| **C** | Tonify the Spleen and augment the Lung. Augment the qi to generate the fluid and nourish the blood. | |
| **D** | • Strongly tonifies the basal qi, the imperial herb for extreme deficiency and collapse of basal qi, mostly used in critical conditions. | • Tonifies the qi of Spleen and Lung, used in place of Ren Shen for moderate or chronic cases of qi deficiency. |

### Ren Shen, Dang Shen, Tai Zi Shen and Xi Yang Shen:

The first three herbs from the list above share a common function of tonifying the Spleen and Lung qi; the strength of their effects decreases in the order from left to right. Xi Yang Shen, the sweet and cold herb, is suitable in deficiency of qi and yin with deficient heat.

### Huang Qi — Bai Zhu — Shan Yao

| | Huang Qi | Bai Zhu | Shan Yao |
|---|---|---|---|
| **C** | Like Dang Shen, these herbs tonify the qi of Spleen and Lung. Combined for mutual reinforcement for patterns of Spleen and Lung qi deficiency. | | |
| **D** | • Strongly tonifies the qi and raises the yang, mostly used for sunken Spleen qi. <br><br>• Promotes the discharge of pus and the generation of tissue. | • Bitter and warm, dries dampness, often used for Spleen deficiency with dampness accumulation. <br><br>• Strengthens the Spleen, augments the qi, and calms the fetus. | • Augments the qi and nourishes the yin, used for Lung and Kidney deficiency with chronic cough or wheezing. <br>• Additional astringing effects to treat leakage of the essence. |
| | • Augment the qi and consolidate the surface, combined for mutual reinforcement to treat unstable protective qi. | | |

## Shan Yao — Huang Jing

|   | Shan Yao | Huang Jing |
|---|----------|------------|
| C | Evenly tonify the qi and yin of Lung, Spleen and Kidney. ||
| D | • Astringent characteristic, used for leakage of the essence, such as Spleen deficiency with diarrhea. | • Relatively stronger in nourishing the yin compared to Shan Yao, not recommended in Spleen deficiency with diarrhea. |

## Shu Di Huang — Dang gui

|   | Shu Di Huang | Dang Gui |
|---|--------------|----------|
| C | Tonify and nourish the blood. Combined for mutual reinforcement in patterns of blood deficiency. ||
| D | • Generates the fluid and augments the marrow for patterns of Kidney yin or essence deficiency.<br>• The imperial herb for nourishing and securing the pre-heaven foundation. | • Tonifies and invigorates the blood for blood deficiency accompanied by blood stasis.<br>• The imperial herb for regulating menstruation and alleviating pain.<br>• Moistens the intestines and unblocks the obstruction of bowel movements. |

## Dang Gui — Bai Shao

|   | Dang Gui | Bai Shao |
|---|----------|----------|
| C | Nourish the yin and blood, and alleviate pain. Combined for mutual reinforcement. ||
| D | • Tonifies the blood.<br>• Invigorates the blood and alleviates pain.<br>• Moistens the intestines and unblocks the obstruction of bowel movements. | • Preserves the yin.<br>• Softens and comforts the Liver and alleviates pain.<br>• Calms and curbs the Liver yang. |

## Dang Gui — E Jiao

|   | Dang Gui | E Jiao |
|---|----------|--------|
| C | Tonify and augment Liver blood. ||
| D | • Also invigorates the blood. | • Also stops bleeding. |

### Sha Shen — Shi Hu — Yu Zhu

|   | Sha Shen | Shi Hu | Yu Zhu |
|---|----------|--------|--------|
| C | Combined for mutual reinforcement. For insufficiency of Lung and Stomach yin and fluid. | | |
| D | • With good strength in nourishing Lung yin. | • Works well in nourishing Stomach yin. <br> • Enhances visual acuity. | • Tonifies without retaining pathogenic factors. |

### Mai Men Dong — Tian Men Dong

|   | Mai Men Dong | Tian Men Dong |
|---|--------------|---------------|
| C | Nourish the yin and moisten dryness. Combined for mutual reinforcement for Lung dryness with cough. | |
| D | • Enters the Heart channel to clear heat from the Heart and eliminate irritability; enters the Stomach channel to augment the Stomach and generate the fluid. | • Extremely cold, has strong effect to clear heat and moisten dryness. <br> • Enters the Kidney channel to nourish Kidney yin. |

### Gui Ban — Bie Jia

|   | Gui Ban | Bie Jia |
|---|---------|---------|
| C | Animal derivatives with direct tonifying effects on the vital substances. Greatly tonify Kidney yin and anchor floating yang. | |
| D | • Stronger in nourishing the yin. <br> • Augments the Kidney and strengthens the bones. | • Stronger in clearing heat. <br> • Softens hardness and dissipates nodules. |

### Nu Zhen Zi — Gou Qi Zi — Sang Shen

|   | Nu Zhen Zi | Gou Qi Zi | Sang Shen |
|---|-----------|-----------|-----------|
| C | Evenly tonify the Liver and Kidney. | | |
| D | • Nourishes the yin only. | • Tonifies the yin and yang. | • Nourishes the yin and blood. |

**Ba Ji Tian, Yin Yang Huo and Xian Mao:**

These three herbs tonify the Kidney and fortify the yang, as well as disperse cold-dampness.

**Rou Cong Rong and Suo Yang:**

These two herbs tonify the Kidney and assist the yang, moisten the intestines and unblock the obstruction of bowel movements.

**Du Zhong, Gou Ji, Xu Duan and Gu Sui Bu:**

These herbs tonify the Liver and Kidney, as well as strengthen or mend the sinews and bones.

**Bu Gu Zhi and Yi Zhi Ren:**

They both tonify the Kidney and assist the yang, secure the essence and restrain leakage.

**Tu Si Zi and Sha Yuan Zi:**

In addition to tonifying the Kidney and securing the essence, they also nourish the Liver and enhance visual acuity.

# HERBS THAT
## Stabilize and Bind 17

Herbs in this category primarily stabilize and bind. Most herbs in this section are sour and astringent. They are effective in restraining the leakage of Lung qi, binding the intestines, astringing the essence, controlling urination and excessive vaginal discharge, stopping bleeding, consolidating the surface and stopping abnormal sweating. They are used for righteous qi deficiency unable to retain essence, such as Lung deficiency with chronic cough, Spleen deficiency with chronic diarrhea, Kidney deficiency with spermatorrhea, Gushing and Leaking Syndromes, excessive vaginal discharge or spontaneous sweating and night sweating.

Most herbs can only treat the branch. In order to treat the branch and root at the same time, these herbs must be combined with herbs that tonify the righteous qi.

The astringent nature of these herbs may retain the pathogenic factors. To prevent such adverse effect, these herbs are not recommended to be used in unresolved exterior conditions, internal dampness accumulation, and constrained heat remaining.

# Wu Wei Zi

*Fructus Schisandrae Chinensis*
*Sour, warm; Heart, Lung, Kidney*

[Characteristics] Possesses all five flavors predominately sour; it is moist despite its warm nature. It primarily restrains and binds, as well as tonifies and augments. Acting on the above it restrains the Lung qi and stops coughing, and on the lower it stabilizes the Kidney and binds the essence. Internally, it restrains the Heart qi and generates the fluid. Externally, it consolidates the protective qi to stop abnormal sweating. It is appropriate for patterns of leakage due to deficiency.

### FUNCTIONS • INDICATIONS & MAJOR COMBINATIONS

### 1. Restrain leakage of Lung qi and nourish the Kidney:
- Lung and Kidney deficiency or Kidney unable to grasp the qi with chronic cough and deficient wheezing. *+ Shan Zhu Yu, Shu Di Huang*
- Cold congested fluids hidden in the Lung with clear copious sputum and unresolved coughing and wheezing. *+ Gan Jiang, Xi Xin*

### 2. Generate the fluid and restrain abnormal sweat:
- Deficiency of the qi and yin with palpitation, shortness of breath, thirst and sweating. *+ Ren Shen, Mai Men Dong*
- Spontaneous sweating or night sweating. *+ Fu Xiao Mai, Mu Li*
- Wasting and Thirsting Disorder. *+ Huang Qi, Tian Hua Fen*

### 3. Bind the essence and stop diarrhea:
- Unstable lower burner with spermatorrhea. *+ Sang Piao Xiao*
- Spleen and Kidney yang deficiency with daybreak diarrhea.
  *+ Rou Dou Kou, Wu Zhu Yu*

### 4. Quiet the Heart and calm the spirit:
- Heart and Kidney yin deficiency with irritability and insomnia.
  *+ Sheng Di Huang, Suan Zao Ren*

### 5. For chronic hepatitis, it can lower the serum level of ALT; administer the powdered form orally.

[Dosage] 3-10 g.

[Comments] As a classic herb in this category, Wu Wei Zi is used for pure deficiency conditions without presence of pathogenic factors. For cold congested fluids hidden in the Lung, combine with Gan Jiang and Xi Xin, acrid and dispersing herbs. With this combination of dispersing and astringing effects, releasing and sealing coexist to treat the complex conditions interdependently.

# Wu Mei

*Fructus Mume*
*Sour, neutral; Liver, Lung, Spleen, Large Intestine*

[Characteristics] Sour and astringent to restrain, and moist texture to generate the fluid, Wu Mei acts on the above to restrain the Lung qi; acts on the lower to bind the intestines; on the middle to generate the fluid and augment the Stomach; it also calms down the roundworms. It is often used for Lung deficiency with chronic cough, insufficient fluid with thirst, Spleen deficiency with chronic diarrhea, and abdominal pain due to roundworms.

| FUNCTIONS • INDICATIONS & MAJOR COMBINATIONS |
|---|
| **1. Restrain the leakage of Lung qi and stop coughing:**<br>• Lung deficiency with chronic cough. *+ E Jiao, Xing Ren* |
| **2. Bind up the intestines and stop diarrhea:**<br>• Unremitting chronic diarrhea. *+ Rou Dou Kou, He Zi* |
| **3. Generate the fluid and alleviate thirst:**<br>• Deficient heat with irritability, intense thirst or Wasting and Thirsting Disorder. *+ Tian Hua Fen, Mai Men Dong* |
| **4. Calm down the roundworms and alleviate pain:**<br>• Severe abdominal pain induced by roundworms. *+ Xi Xin, Huang Lian* |
| **5. Treat bleeding for Gushing and Leaking Syndromes when taken orally; for toxic abscesses, apply topically.** |

[Dosage] 3-10 g. May use up to 30 g. Charred form to stop diarrhea and stop bleeding; for topical application, grind the herb or powder the charred form.

[Precautions] Not recommended for use in unresolved exterior condition and internal excess heat accumulation.

# Fu Xiao Mai

*Fructus Tritici Levis Immaturus*
*Sweet, cool; Heart*

[Characteristics] Sweet and cool to augment the qi and eliminate heat, Fu Xiao Mai primarily enters the Heart channel. It is the primary herb used to stop sweating and is appropriate for all patterns of deficient sweating.

### FUNCTIONS • INDICATIONS & MAJOR COMBINATIONS

**Augment the qi, eliminate heat and stop abnormal sweating:**
- Qi deficiency with spontaneous sweating. *+ Huang Qi*
- Yin deficiency with night sweating. *+ Wu Wei Zi, Bai Shao*

[Dosage] 15-30 g.

[Comments] "Sweat is the fluid of the Heart." Mainly entering the Heart channel, and characterized by its nature of sweet and cool, Fu Xiao Mai stops sweating by augmenting the qi and eliminating heat; it does not inhibit the excretion of sweat.

[Addendum]
**Xiao Mai**
*Fructus Tritici Levis*
Sweet and cool, it enters the Heart channel. Xiao Mai, nourishes the Heart and eliminates irritability. It is used to treat Restless Organ Disorder. 30-60 g.

# Ma Huang Gen

*Radix Ephedrae*
*Sweet, neutral; Lung*

[Characteristics] It exclusively restrains the sweat for all patterns of deficiency.

### FUNCTIONS • INDICATIONS & MAJOR COMBINATIONS

**Stop sweating:**
- Qi deficiency with spontaneous sweating. *+ Huang Qi, Bai Zhu*
- Yin deficiency with night sweating. *+ Sheng Di Huang, Mu Li*

[Dosage] 3-10 g.

[Precautions] Contraindicated in exterior conditions.

[Comments] Coming from the same plant, Ma Huang Gen specifically stops sweating; while Ma Huang, a powerful diaphoretic, does just the opposite.

# Chun Pi  *o~ Chun Gen Pi*

*Cortex Ailanthi*
*Bitter, astringent, cold; Large Intestine, ~~Stomach~~* L i v

[Characteristics] Bitter and cold to clear heat and dry dampness, Chun Pi is an astringent herb that restrains and binds. It enters the Large Intestine to stop diarrhea and it enters the Liver channel to cool the blood and stop bleeding.

**FUNCTIONS • INDICATIONS & MAJOR COMBINATIONS**

**1. Clear heat, dry dampness, bind up the intestines and astringe excessive vaginal discharge:**
   - Chronic diarrhea and dysentery disorder or bloody stool. *+ He Zi*
   - Damp-heat with excessive vaginal discharge. *+ Huang Bai*

**2. Cool the blood and stop bleeding:**
   - Heat in the blood with heavy menstruation or unremitting Gushing and Leaking Syndromes. *+ Gui Ban, Xiang Fu*

**3. Kill parasites and alleviate itchiness for skin disorders related to fungal infection with itchiness and discharge; use as an external wash.**

[Dosage] 3-10 g.


# He Zi

*Fructus Chebulae*
*Bitter, sour, astringent, neutral; Lung, Large Intestine*

[Characteristics] Bitter in nature, it descends the qi; it also has an astringing effect. Raw form enters the Lung to restrain Lung qi and benefit the throat; roasted form enters the intestines to stop diarrhea.

**FUNCTIONS • INDICATIONS & MAJOR COMBINATIONS**

**1. Bind up the intestines and stop diarrhea:**
   - Chronic diarrhea, chronic dysentery disorder and rectal prolapse.
     *+ Gan Jiang, Chen Pi*

**2. Restrain the leakage of Lung qi and benefit the throat:**
   - Chronic cough and loss of voice. *+ Jie Geng, Gan Cao*

[Dosage] 3-10 g. Raw to restrain the Lung qi; roasted to stop diarrhea.

[Precautions] Contraindicated in unresolved exterior condition or internal damp-heat accumulation.

# Rou Dou Kou

*Semen Myristicae*
*Acrid, warm; Spleen, Stomach, Large Intestine*

[Characteristics] Drying and astringing, Rou Dou Kou primarily binds the intestines and stops diarrhea. It is also acrid, warm and aromatic in nature; it warms the Spleen and Stomach and facilitates the movement of qi.

**FUNCTIONS • INDICATIONS & MAJOR COMBINATIONS**

### 1. Bind up the intestines and stop diarrhea:
- Spleen and Kidney yang deficiency with daybreak diarrhea.
  *+ Wu Wei Zi, Wu Zhu Yu*

### 2. Warm the middle burner and move the qi:
- Congealed cold and stagnant qi with distention and pain in the epigastrium and abdomen, lack of appetite and vomiting. *+ Xiang Fu, Gao Liang Jiang*

[Dosage] 3-10 g. To enhance the effects of warming the middle and stopping diarrhea, it is recommended to use the defatty form.

[Precautions] Contraindicated in damp-heat dysentery.

# Chi Shi Zhi

*Halloysitum Rubrum*
*Sweet, sour, astringent, warm; Stomach, Large Intestine*

[Characteristics] It exclusively restrains and binds, primarily used to bind the intestines and stop diarrhea, as well as stop bleeding. Topical application can promote healing and generate the tissue.

**FUNCTIONS • INDICATIONS & MAJOR COMBINATIONS**

### 1. Bind up the intestines and stop diarrhea:
- Incontinence of bowel movements. *+ Yu Yu Liang*

### 2. Stop bleeding:
- Gushing and Leaking Syndromes. *+ Ce Bai Ye, Hai Piao Xiao*

### 3. Promote healing and generate the tissue, used for topical application.

[Dosage] 10-20 g.

[Precautions] Not recommended in pregnancy. Contraindicated in damp-heat.

# Shan Zhu Yu

*Fructus Corni*
*Sour, slightly warm; Liver, Kidney*

[Characteristics] Sour, astringent and slightly warm, Shan Zu Yu primarily enters the Liver and Kidney channels. It restrains to bind the essence and qi; it tonifies the Liver and Kidney to nourish the essence, blood and basal yang. It is the imperial herb that tonifies the Kidney and binds the essence. With the appropriate combinations, it treats all patterns of Kidney and Liver deficiency and instability of the lower burner.

| FUNCTIONS • INDICATIONS & MAJOR COMBINATIONS |
|---|
| **1. Tonify and augment the Liver and Kidney:** <br> • Liver and Kidney deficiency with dizziness, vertigo, soreness and weakness of the lower back and knees. *+ Shu Di Huang, Shan Yao* <br> • Kidney yang insufficiency with soreness and weakness of the lower back and knees. *+ Fu Zi, Rou Gui* |
| **2. Stabilize and bind:** <br> • Kidney deficiency with spermatorrhea and nocturnal emission. *+ Sha Yuan Zi, Qian Shi* <br> • Urinary incontinence. *+ Sang Piao Xiao, Fu Peng Zi* <br> • General weakness with unremitting deficient sweating. *+ Ren Shen, Mu Li* <br> • Unstable Penetrating and Conception vessels with heavy menstruation or Gushing and Leaking Syndromes. *+ Huang Qi, Hai Piao Xiao* |

[Dosage] 6-15 g. May use up to 30 g.

[Precautions] Not recommended for yin deficiency with heat, damp-heat and urinary dysfunction.

[Comments] The alternative name is Zao Pi.

# Jin Ying Zi

*Fructus Rosae Laevigatae*
*Sour, astringent, neutral; Kidney, Bladder, Large Intestine*

[Characteristics] It exclusively restrains and binds without any tonifying ability. Jing Ying Zi treats all patterns of deficiency with the presence of unstable lower burner.

**FUNCTIONS • INDICATIONS & MAJOR COMBINATIONS**

**1. Stabilize the Kidney and bind the essence:**
- Lower burner deficiency and instability with spermatorrhea, urinary incontinence and excessive vaginal discharge. *+ Qian Shi*

**2. Bind the intestines and stop diarrhea:**
- Chronic diarrhea or dysentery disorder. *+ Dang Shen, Shan Yao*

[Dosage] 6-20 g. May simmer to syrup consistency for oral administration.

[Precautions] Not recommended for conditions of excess pathogenic factors.


# Qian Shi

*Semen Euryales*
*Sweet, astringent, neutral; Spleen, Kidney*

[Characteristics] Sweet and astringent, Qian Shi enters the Spleen and Kidney channels. It has the functions of strengthening the Spleen to stop diarrhea, and augmenting the Kidney to bind the essence, with emphasis on the latter function. It treats all patterns of Spleen and Kidney deficiency and instability.

**FUNCTIONS • INDICATIONS & MAJOR COMBINATIONS**

**1. Augment the Kidney and bind the essence:**
- Kidney deficiency with nocturnal emission, premature ejaculation and spermatorrhea. *+ Sha Yuan Zi, Lian Zi*
- Kidney deficiency with frequent urination and excessive vaginal discharge. *+ Jin Ying Zi*
- Damp-heat with excessive vaginal discharge. *+ Che Qian Zi, Huang Bai*

**2. Strengthen the Spleen and stop diarrhea:**
- Spleen deficiency with chronic diarrhea. *+ Bai Zhu, Shan Yao*

[Dosage] 10-15 g.

# Lian Zi

*Semen Nelumbinis*
*Sweet, astringent, neutral; Heart, Spleen, Kidney*

[Characteristics] With similar effects to Qian Shi, combined for mutual reinforcement, Lian Zi has a stronger effect to strengthen the Spleen to stop diarrhea. It also nourishes the Heart and calms the spirit for deficient irritability and insomnia.

**FUNCTIONS • INDICATIONS & MAJOR COMBINATIONS**

### 1. Strengthen the Spleen and stop diarrhea:
- Spleen deficiency with chronic diarrhea. *+ Bai Zhu, Shan Yao*

### 2. Augment the Kidney and bind the essence:
- Kidney deficiency with nocturnal emission, premature ejaculation and spermatorrhea. *+ Sha Yuan Zi, Qian Shi*
- Spleen deficiency with excessive vaginal discharge. *+ Shan Yao*

### 3. Nourish the Heart and calm the spirit:
- Heart deficiency with irritability, palpitation, agitation and insomnia. *+ Mai Men Dong, Fu Shen*

[Dosage] 6-15 g.

[Precautions] Not recommended for use in constipation.

[Comments] Lian Zi is the mature seed of lotus; herbs from the same plant are:

    **Lian Xu**, the stamen of lotus, with the same properties as Lian Zi, effectively stabilizes the Kidney and binds the essence; it is primarily used for nocturnal emission, frequent urination and excessive vaginal discharge.

    **Lian Fang**, the mature receptacle of lotus, bitter, astringent and cold, has the effects to stop hemorrhaging and transform stasis for Gushing and Leaking Syndromes, hematuria and bleeding hemorrhoid.

    **Lian Zi Xin**, the newly grown plumule, bitter and cold, enters the Heart channel to drain fire for Warm-Febrile Disease with fever, irritability and loss of consciousness. It also treats heat in the blood with hematemesis.

## [Addendum]
## He Ye
*Folium Nelumbinis*

Bitter, astringent and neutral, it relieves summerheat and drains dampness, lifts yang qi and stops bleeding. It is used to treat all conditions due to summerheat accompanied by dampness and Spleen deficiency with diarrhea, and is also used to treat patterns of bleeding. 3-10 g.

       **Herbs that Stabilize and Bind**

# Sang Piao Xiao

*Ootheca Mantidis*
*Sweet, salty, neutral; Kidney, Liver*

[Characteristics] Assists the yang to restrain and bind the essence. It treats Kidney deficiency unable to bind the essence with enuresis and frequent urination.

**Tonify the Kidney, assist the yang and bind the essence:**
- Kidney yang deficiency with lower burner deficient cold.
  — Impotence and premature ejaculation. *+ Lu Rong, Ba Ji Tian*
  — Enuresis and frequent urination. *+ Yuan Zhi, Long Gu*

[Dosage] 3-10 g.

[Precautions] Contraindicated for deficient heat and heat in the Bladder.

# Hai Piao Xiao

*Endoconcha Sepiae*
*Salty, astringent, slightly warm; Kidney, Liver*

[Characteristics] It exclusively restrains and binds without any tonifying ability. It is especially effective in astringing to stop bleeding, restraining and binding the essence, and reducing acidity.

**1. Astringe and stop bleeding:**
- Gushing and Leaking Syndromes. *+ Qian Cao Gen*
- Lung and Stomach bleeding. *+ Bai Ji*

**2. Bind the essence and astringe excessive vaginal discharge:**
- Cold or heat type of excessive vaginal discharge. *+ Bai Zhi*
- Nocturnal emission. *+ Shan Zhu Yu, Sha Yuan Zi*

**3. Reduce acidity and alleviate pain:**
- Stomach upset and acid regurgitation. *+ Bei Mu, Bai Ji*

**4. Resolve dampness and promote healing, often applied topically.**

[Dosage] 6-10 g. Reduce to 1.5-3 g. when using the powdered form.

[Precautions] Not recommended for use in yin deficiency with heat.

[Comments] The alternative name is Wu Zei Gu.

# Bai Guo

*Semen Ginkgo*
*Sweet, bitter, astringent, neutral, slightly toxic; Lung*

[Characteristics] Astringent to restrain leakage and bitter to dry dampness, Bai Guo acts on the above to restrain Lung qi and stop wheezing, and on the lower to eliminate dampness and stop excessive vaginal discharge. Neutral in nature, it treats either cold or heat pattern.

**FUNCTIONS • INDICATIONS & MAJOR COMBINATIONS**

**1. Restrain the leakage of Lung qi and stop wheezing:**
- Wind-cold wheezing and coughing up copious sputum.
  *+ Ma Huang, Gan Cao*
- Phlegm-heat with coughing and wheezing. *+ Ma Huang, Sang Bai Pi*

**2. Eliminate dampness and stop excessive vaginal discharge:**
- Cold patterns of excessive vaginal discharge with thin watery consistency. *+ Lian Zi, Hu Jiao*
- Heat patterns of excessive vaginal discharge with turbid yellow consistency and foul odor. *+ Huang Bai, Qian Shi*
- Cloudy urination. *+ Bi Xie, Yi Zhi Ren*

[Dosage] 6-10 g.

[Precautions] Slightly toxic, raw herb or large dose may cause intoxication. Not recommended for cough with viscous sputum that is difficult to expectorate.

[Comments] ❶ The alternative name is Yin Xing.

❷ Bai Guo restrains Lung qi to stop wheezing, and is commonly combined with Ma Huang. Ma Huang disperses Lung qi; Bai Guo restrains Lung qi and transforms phlegm. In this combination, one disperses while the other restrains to enhance the effects of calming wheezing; Bai Guo can also prevent leakage of Lung qi. In traditional textbooks, Bai Guo is usually classified into herbs that transform phlegm and stop coughing.

[Addendum]
**Yin Xing Ye**
*Folium Ginkgo*

With the same properties and entering the same channels as Bai Guo, it restrains Lung qi to calm wheezing, as well as alleviates pain. It is used for Lung deficiency with cough and wheezing. Currently, it is used in the cases of cerebral, cardiac vascular disorders, such as hypertension, coronary arterial disease, angina, etc.

## [Remarks & Differentiations]

**Wu Wei Zi, Wu Mei, He Zi and Bai Guo:**
All of these herbs restrain the leakage of Lung qi.

**Fu Xiao Mai, Ma Huang Gen and Wu Wei Zi:**
These herbs share the common effect to astringe and restrain abnormal sweat.

**Wu Wei Zi, Wu Mei, Chun Pi, He Zi, Rou Dou Kou and Chi Shi Zhi:**
All are capable of binding up the intestines and stopping diarrhea.

**Shan Zhu Yu, Jin Ying Zi, Qian Shi, Lian Zi, Sang Piao Xiao and Hai Piao Xiao:**
Primarily augment the Kidney and bind the essence.

### Fu Xiao Mai — Ma Huang Gen

|   | Fu Xiao Mai | Ma Huang Gen |
|---|---|---|
| C | Stop abnormal sweating; treat spontaneous sweating and night sweating. Commonly combined for mutual reinforcement. | |
| D | • Sweet and cold to augment qi, eliminate heat and stop abnormal sweating. | • Astringent to exclusively restrain abnormal sweat. |

### Qian Shi — Lian Zi

|   | Qian Shi | Lian Zi |
|---|---|---|
| C | Strengthen the Spleen and stop diarrhea. Augment the Kidney and bind the essence. Commonly combined for mutual reinforcement. | |
| D | • Stronger in augmenting the Kidney and binding the essence. | • Stronger in strengthening the Spleen and stopping diarrhea.<br>• Also enters the Heart channel to nourish the Heart and calm the spirit. |

## Sang Piao Xiao — Hai Piao Xiao

| | **Sang Piao Xiao** | **Hai Piao Xiao** |
|---|---|---|
| **C** | Augment the Kidney and bind the essence. | |
| **D** | • Assists Kidney yang to restrain and bind the essence. Astringes while tonifies. | • Exclusively restrains without having any tonifying effects.<br><br>• Astringes and stops bleeding.<br>• Reduces acidity and alleviates pain.<br>• Resolves dampness and promotes the healing of sores. |

# HERBS THAT
## Expel Parasites 18

These herbs eradicate and/or kill parasites. They are used for treating cases of roundworms, pinworms, hookworms and tapeworms. Clinical manifestations include indigestion, pain around the umbilicus, pica and sallow complexion.

According to various types of intestinal parasites, select the appropriate herbs for the best result. Usually, these herbs are combined with herbs that strengthen the Spleen.

These herbs should be taken on an empty stomach. Some herbs are toxic; refer to individual dosage prior to application. Use these herbs with caution in pregnant women, elderly and those with general weakness.

# Shi Jun Zi

*Fructus Quisqualis*
***Sweet, warm; Spleen, Stomach***

**[Characteristics]** Shi Jun Zi is sweet and warm, augments the Spleen and Stomach, and is the primary herb for eradicating roundworms. It also has a pleasant taste and smell, easy to take.

**FUNCTIONS • INDICATIONS & MAJOR COMBINATIONS**

**1. Kill parasites:**
- For mild cases of roundworms, stir-fry this herb alone until the aroma is present and take orally. For severe cases, *+ Ku Lian Pi, Bing Lang*

**2. Reduce accumulations and strengthen the Spleen:**
- Childhood indigestion with emaciation, sallow complexion and distended abdomen. *+ Dang Shen, Bing Lang*

**[Dosage]** 6-10 g. Stir-fry until the aroma is present and take orally. For children, take 1.5 piece/age throughout the day and not to exceed 20 pieces/day.

**[Precautions]** Dizziness and vomiting may occur when taken with tea or from overdose. Discontinuing the herb can relieve those symptoms.

# Ku Lian Pi

*Cortex Meliae*
***Bitter, cold, toxic; Spleen, Stomach, Liver***

**[Characteristics]** Compared with Shi Jun Zi, Ku Lian Pi has a much stronger effect in eradicating parasites; however, because of its toxic nature, it should be used with caution. It can clear heat and dry dampness to alleviate itchiness from tinea.

**FUNCTIONS • INDICATIONS & MAJOR COMBINATIONS**

**1. Kill parasites:**
- Roundworms, pinworms and hookworms. *+ Shi Jun Zi*

**2. Dry dampness:**
- For tinea of the head and body, use the decoction as an external wash.

**[Dosage]** 6-15 g. 15-30 g. if using the fresh herb.

**[Precautions]** Toxic, not to exceed the recommended dose. Contraindicated in hepatic disorders.

# Bing Lang   Betel Nut

*Semen Arecae*
*Acrid, bitter, warm; Stomach, Large Intestine*

[Characteristics] It has a strong effect in eradicating various intestinal parasites. Acrid to disperse and bitter to descend, Bing Lang facilitates the movement of qi and reduces the accumulations to treat abdominal distention due to food retention; it also promotes urination to treat edema.

| FUNCTIONS • INDICATIONS & MAJOR COMBINATIONS |
| --- |
| **1. Kill parasites:**<br>  • Accumulations of various intestinal parasites, especially for tapeworms with abdominal pain. *+ Nan Gua Zi* |
| **2. Regulate the movement of qi and reduce accumulations:**<br>  • Food retention and qi stagnation with abdominal distention. *+ Mai Ya, Shen Qu*<br>  • Food retention generating heat with constipation or dysentery disorders with tenesmus. *+ Mu Xiang, Da Huang* |
| **3. Promote urination and reduce edema:**<br>  • Excess patterns of edema. *+ Ze Xie, Shang Lu* |
| **4. Malarial disorders.** |

[Dosage] 6-15 g. May increase dose to 60-120 g when used alone to expel tapeworms.

[Addendum]
**Da Fu Pi**   Betel Nut Peel (hull)
*Pericarpium Arecae*
Acrid and slightly warm, it enters the Spleen, Stomach, Large Intestine and Small Intestine channels. It descends the flow of qi, expands the middle burner, promotes urination and reduces edema for qi stagnation with distention in the epigastrium and abdomen, and for systemic edema.

**Herbs that Expel Parasites**

# HERBS THAT
## Are Applied Topically 19

Introduced in this chapter are herbs primarily to be applied topically. Herbs in this category relieve toxicity, dissipate nodules, kill parasites and alleviate itchiness. Modify the prescription based on the clinical manifestations and locations of the disorders. Some herbs can also be taken internally.

Most of these herbs are toxic. Although they are applied topically, they are not to be used on large area or for long periods of time. When prescribing it for oral administration, follow the dosage guidelines strictly and prepare them in pill or powdered form.

# Liu Huang

*Sulfur*
*Sour, warm, toxic; Kidney, Large Intestine*

**[Characteristics]** Warm and drying to relieve toxicity, it kills parasites and alleviates itchiness when applied externally. Entering the Kidney, it tonifies the fire in the Gate of Vitality and assists the Kidney to grasp the qi when taken orally.

**FUNCTIONS • INDICATIONS & MAJOR COMBINATIONS**

**1. Kill parasites and stop itchiness:**
  • For scabies and eczema, apply the mixture of powdered form with sesame oil or use it to moxa on the topical lesions.

**2. Tonify the fire and assist the yang:**
  • Insufficient Kidney yang with impotence. *+ Lu Rong, Bu Gu Zhi*
  • Kidney unable to grasp the qi with wheezing. *+ Fu Zi, Rou Gui*

**[Dosage]** 1-3 g. add to pills; modify dose for external use accordingly.

**[Precautions]** Contraindicated during pregnancy.

# Bai Fan

*Alumen*
*Sour, astringent, cold; Lung, Liver, Spleen, Stomach, Large Intestine*

**[Characteristics]** Bai Fan, internally, transforms phlegm, stops bleeding and diarrhea; it becomes drying and astringent after it is processed into calcined form and is applied topically to absorb dampness, stop itchiness and kill parasites.

**FUNCTIONS • INDICATIONS & MAJOR COMBINATIONS**

**1. Dry dampness and stop itchiness:**
  • Scabies and eczema with itchiness, apply topically. *+ Duan Shi Gao*

**2. Stop bleeding and alleviate diarrhea:**
  • Hematemesis, subcutaneous and mucosa bleeding and traumatic hemorrhaging, take orally or apply topically. *+ Er Cha*
  • Chronic diarrhea and chronic dysentery disorder. *+ Wu Bei Zi, He Zi*

**3. Clear heat and transform phlegm for seizures and manic behaviors.**

**[Dosage]** 1-3 g. add to pills; modify dose for external use accordingly.

**[Comments]** The alternative name is Ming Fan.

# She Chuang Zi

*Fructus Cnidii*
*Acrid, bitter, warm; Kidney*

[Characteristics] External wash with the decoction is an effective method to dry dampness and alleviate itchiness. It also warms the Kidney and fortifies the yang.

| FUNCTIONS • INDICATIONS & MAJOR COMBINATIONS |
|---|
| **1. Dry dampness, eradicate parasites and alleviate itchiness:**<br>• Eczema or scabies with severe itchiness, wash with the decoction.<br>*+ Ku Shen, Huang Bai* |
| **2. Warm the Kidney and fortify the yang:**<br>• Impotence or infertility due to cold womb. *+ Wu Wei Zi, Tu Si Zi* |
| **3. Disperse cold and dispel wind:**<br>• Dampness-type of Painful Obstruction with lower back pain.<br>*+ Du Zhong, Sang Ji Sheng* |

[Dosage] 3-10 g. 15-30 g. when applied topically.

[Precautions] Not recommended to administer orally in yin deficiency with heat or damp-heat in the lower burner.


# Lu Feng Fang

*Nidus Vespae*
*Sweet, neutral, toxic; Stomach*

[Characteristics] Lu Feng Fang's toxic nature can be used to fight the toxins in the body; it also dispels wind, unblocks the painful obstruction and alleviates pain.

| FUNCTIONS • INDICATIONS & MAJOR COMBINATIONS |
|---|
| **1. Attack toxins and eradicate parasites:**<br>• Carbuncles, gangrene and scrofula, roast the herb until it turns yellow, then powder it for oral administration, or apply the decoction as an external wash. |
| **2. Dispel wind:**<br>• Wind-cold-damp Painful Obstruction. *+ Gui Zhi, Wu Tou* |

[Dosage] 6-10 g. or 1.5-3 g when using the powdered form.

[Precautions] Not recommended for deficient conditions.

**Herbs that are Applied Topically**

# List by Pinyin Names

**List by Pinyin Names**

# *Index of Latin Pharmaceutical Names*

# *Chinese Pathological Terminology*

# *Bibliography*

*Physicians' desk reference* (2000). (vol. 1). Beijing: Chemical Industry Press.

He, X. et. al. (1998). *Zhongyaoxue* [The Chinese materia medica]. Beijing: Academic Press.

Jiangsu New Medical School. (1975). *Zhongyao dacidian* [Chinese herbal dictionary]. Shanghai: Shanghai People's Publishing House.

Ling, Y. et. al. (1984). *Zhongyaoxue* [Materia medica]. Shanghai: Shanghai Science and Technology Press.

Weng, W. et. al. (1983). *Zhongyao jianbie yingyong* [Chinese herbal differentiation and application]. Beijing: Beijing University of Traditional Chinese Medicine.

Zeng, D. et. al. (1987). *Zhongyiyao zhuticibiao* [Subject headings for traditional Chinese medicine]. Beijing: Beijing Science and Technology Press.

Zeng, D. et. al. (1990). Zhongyiyaoxue [Chinese medicine]. In *Zhongguo baike dacidian*. Beijing: Huaxia Publishing House.


Bensky, D. & Gamble, A. (1993). *Chinese herbal medicine: Materia medica.* (2nd ed.). Seattle, WA: Eastland Press.

Thomas, C. L. (Ed.). (1989). *Taber's cyclopedic medical dictionary.* (16th ed.). Philadelphia, PA: F. A. Davis.

Wiseman, N. & Ye, F. (1999). *A practical dictionary of Chinese medicine.* (2nd ed.). Brookline, MA: Paradigm Publications.